Praise for *Full*

Asheritah beautifully lays out a spiritual battle plan for those struggling over a fixation with food. *Full* is the reminder that your soul was made to crave God above all else!

Lysa TerKeurst
New York Times bestselling author and president of Proverbs 31 Ministries

Food is both a great gift from our good Creator and a terrible taskmaster that keeps many of us in perpetual bondage. Asheritah invites us to break free from food fixation, to honor God and enjoy Him in our food choices, and to find true satisfaction in the fullness of His grace.

Nancy DeMoss Wolgemuth
Author, teacher/host of *Revive Our Hearts*

It just takes a few paragraphs to sense that Asheritah is a friend. I saw myself in her stories and I think you will too. This book will help you become more aware of your relationship with food while driving you closer to Jesus, the true Bread of Life.

Arlene Pellicane
Coauthor of *Growing Up Social: Raising Relational Kids in a Screen-Driven World*

"Wow. She really gets it." Page after page, I spoke those words aloud as I read this important book. If you have ever struggled with food, this book is for you. In *Full*, Asheritah thoroughly dismantles the lies we believe about food—and about ourselves—and then points us straight to the truth we find in Jesus. This book will set a lot of women free, and it will stir up within them a holy hunger.

Jennifer Dukes Lee
Author of *The Happiness Dare*

Equal parts practical and inspiring, Asheritah Ciuciu balances the perfect blend of soulful encouragement and real-life application. Diving straight into the heart of the matter, *Full* is a book any woman who has struggled with a food fixation needs to read.

RUTH SOUKUP
New York Times bestselling author of *Living Well Spending Less* and *Unstuffed*

This is not a simple book on how to eat right and lose weight. Asheritah's fine research into the psychology of food fixation and the biblical and spiritual roots of this preoccupation is captivating. But she doesn't stop there. She surveys the biblical perspective of God's gift of food and how to celebrate and serve others with food. An incredibly uplifting and hope-filled book.

WILLIAM E. BROWN
Senior Fellow for Worldview and Culture, the Colson Center for Christian Worldview

This book isn't only about food; it's also about worship. *Full* is a refreshing guidebook to help reframe your relationship with food as you draw closer to God. With practical solutions and gentle encouragement, Asheritah reminds us of this truth: food is a gift, and worship happens around a table.

DEIDRA RIGGS
Author of *Every Little Thing* and *One: Unity in a Divided World*

After reading *Full*, I am convinced that it is a vital resource for all Christian counselors to help individuals and groups break free from food fixation and grow deeper in their walk with Christ. Asheritah compels readers to explore and uncover the spiritual and emotional roots of food fixation while also providing practical application steps toward health and wholeness. *Full* is refreshingly honest and compassionately convicting, addressing a topic that I have yet to hear preached from the pulpit in twenty-plus years of regular church attendance and yet one that every soul is hungry to hear.

ANN MARIE APONTE
The Professional Counseling Group

If your relationship with food has been a battlefield for you, and if you would like to take a biblical approach in pursuing victory, then you should hit pause on your diet while embracing the mindset shift Asheritah unpacks in *Full*.

ELISA PULLIAM
Author of *Meet the New You: A 21-Day Plan for Embracing Fresh Attitudes and Focused Habits for Real Life Change*; owner of KaleoAgency.net

Full is the perfect blend of scriptural truths and practical applications exposing the mental battle we are engaged in. Going beyond food fixations, Asheritah teaches us to embrace the truth and transforming power found in God's Word. Christian women need the encouragement so carefully penned here. I am so thankful Asheritah wrote *Full* and grateful for the battle plan found within the pages of this book.

YUKIKO JOHNSON
Women's Ministries Coordinator, First Baptist Church, Minot, ND

Every now and again a woman is brave enough to shine the light, full and revealing, into the darkest recesses of her own heart, with the hope of illuminating the same sin-tendencies bound up in the murky corners of other people's private lives. That is what Asheritah Ciuciu has done in the pages of *Full*. As readers follow along on her journey to understand each misplaced craving, they can't help but come face to face with the only one who can ever truly satisfy their own deep hunger!

WENDY SPEAKE BRUNNER
Coauthor of *Triggers* and *Life Creative*

This book is a must-read for all those eager to break the chains of food fixation once and for all. Embark with Asheritah on a life-transforming journey from guilt, shame, and defeat to the freedom of finding true, sustaining satisfaction in God.

MICHELLE DERUSHA
Author of *50 Women Every Christian Should Know* and *Spiritual Misfit: A Memoir of Uneasy Faith*

If you struggle with food fixation as I do, *Full* is a must-read. It's vulnerably written, wonderfully practical, and it clearly points to the one who will always satisfy us more than our favorite comfort food.

ASHLEIGH SLATER
Author of *Team Us*

Through Scripture, practical encouragement, and personal experience, Asheritah will lead you on a journey toward the true satisfaction, deep contentment, and lasting freedom that can only be found in Jesus. You will not regret reading this book.

ERIKA DAWSON
Writer/blogger at erikadawson.com

I can't wait until this book comes out. It is so timely for me right now. I have oodles of "diet books" and food-focused devotionals on my shelves, but Asheritah's book has real "meat" to help me deal with food fixation. Love it and will be buying some as gifts.

DAWN WILSON
Blogger; research assistant for Revive Our Hearts/Nancy DeMoss Wolgemuth

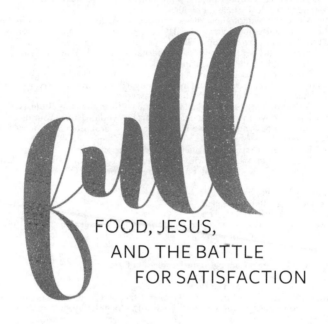

full

FOOD, JESUS, AND THE BATTLE FOR SATISFACTION

ASHERITAH CIUCIU

MOODY PUBLISHERS

CHICAGO

All Scripture quotations, unless otherwise indicated, are taken from the Holy Bible, New International Version®, NIV®. Copyright © 1973, 1978, 1984, 2011 by Biblica, Inc.™ Used by permission of Zondervan. All rights reserved worldwide. www.zondervan.com. The "NIV" and "New International Version" are trademarks registered in the United States Patent and Trademark Office by Biblica, Inc.™

Scripture quotations marked ESV are from The Holy Bible, English Standard Version® (ESV®), copyright © 2001 by Crossway, a publishing ministry of Good News Publishers. Used by permission. All rights reserved.

Scripture quotations marked NLT are taken from the Holy Bible, New Living Translation, copyright © 1996, 2004, 2007, 2013 by Tyndale House Foundation. Used by permission of Tyndale House Publishers, Inc., Carol Stream, Illinois 60188. All rights reserved.

Emphasis to Scripture has been added by the author.

Published in association with Literary Agent Tawny Johnson of D.C. Jacobson and Associates LLC, 537 SE Ash Street, Suite 203, Portland, OR 97214.

Edited by Pam Pugh
Interior design: Ragont Design
Cover design: Erik M. Peterson
Cover image of raspberries copyright © 2015 by Jeff Wasserman / Stocksy (692078)
Author photo: Ashley McComb

Library of Congress Cataloging-in-Publication Data

Names: Ciuciu, Asheritah, author.
Title: Full : food, Jesus, and the battle for satisfaction / Asheritah Ciuciu.
Description: Chicago : Moody Publishers, 2017. | Includes bibliographical
   references.
Identifiers: LCCN 2016035754 (print) | LCCN 2016046425 (ebook) | ISBN
   9780802415370 | ISBN 9780802495297
Subjects: LCSH: Food--Religious aspects--Christianity. | Habit
   breaking--Religious aspects--Christianity. | Spiritual life--Christianity.
   | Satisfaction--Religious aspects--Christianity. | Contentment--Religious
   aspects--Christianity.
Classification: LCC BR115.N87 C58 2017 (print) | LCC BR115.N87 (ebook) | DDC
   241/.68--dc23
LC record available at https://lccn.loc.gov/2016035754

All information stated in this book is for information purposes only. The information is not specific medical advice for any individual. The content of this book should not substitute medical advice from a health professional. If you have a health problem, speak to your doctor or a health professional immediately about your condition.

We hope you enjoy this book from Moody Publishers. Our goal is to provide high-quality, thought-provoking books and products that connect truth to your real needs and challenges. For more information on other books and products written and produced from a biblical perspective, go to www.moodypublishers.com or write to:

Moody Publishers
820 N. LaSalle Boulevard
Chicago, IL 60610

5 7 9 10 8 6 4

Printed in the United States of America

To Jesus Christ, the Bread of Life,
who is teaching me each day to feast on Him
while also enjoying a warm croissant now and then.

And to my handsome man, who journeyed with
me through every high and low written on these pages
and cheered me on just the same: *Te iubesc*.

Contents

Foreword

What do you expect from a book with a title like *Full*? I opened the pages and smiled as I read the dedication:

> *To Jesus Christ, the Bread of Life, who is teaching me each day to feast on Him while enjoying a warm croissant now and then.*

This dedication made me want to read *Full*—it offered humor and balance! Let me assure you that it is not another diet book or a healthy-eating plan. You will find no recipes or swapping recommended here. Why not? Because Asheritah knew *what* and *how* to eat but, when faced with her favorite comfort foods, lost all willpower to eat healthfully. Food had ungodly control over her, and no number of rules was going to change that.

I can relate. I told a nutritionist once that there just is no comfort in carrots. I got a strange look back. But it's the truth! I tried every eating plan, believed promises . . . *If you eat this way for eight weeks, you'll never want to go back to carbs and cake.* Wrong. Bingeing and yo-yo dieting create havoc and produce very temporary results. So what do you do? Just throw out the scale and give up? And eat all the potato chips you crave?

Asheritah has a better, more creative answer. The yo-yo eating, grasping on to every new diet for a week and then giving up, will never work because the paradigm is all wrong. Our problem is not what we eat but why we seek fullness in something that will never satisfy. So what did this lovely young

Romanian American woman do to change her paradigm?

"I stopped praying for a smaller waist and faster metabolism and began praying, *Deeper Lord. Take me deeper into your presence.*"

John Piper agrees with Asheritah's shift in her thinking. "If you don't feel strong desires for the manifestation of God, it is not because you have drunk deeply and are satisfied. It is because you have nibbled so long at the table of the world. Your soul is stuffed with small things and there is no room for the great God. God did not create you for this. There is an appetite for God. And it can be awakened."

I was excited! A book I thought would teach me how to eat right was really going to take me by the hand and show me how to awaken a deeper desire for my God. And in the process of being filled up with Him, I would naturally desire to be filled up with the right foods—in sensible amounts.

Sound too good to be true? Well then, you should just read this special book for yourself. I'm so glad I did. I learned things about my food triggers that I didn't know. But more importantly, my heart was stirred to run after our great God.

Friend, follow my example and keep turning these pages. I promise you will be grateful you did!

LINDA DILLOW

Author of *Calm My Anxious Heart, Satisfy My Thirsty Soul,* and coauthor of *Surprised by the Healer*

Let's Get Started

For a brief moment, I was convinced some desperate sugar-bingeing alien had possessed me.

On my daughter's first birthday, as our guests were leaving and family was helping tear down the party decorations, I ate a slice of cake. Why not? It had been a stressful day. Make that a stressful couple of weeks. Determined to give my baby the best *Very Hungry Caterpillar* birthday party ever, I had spent late nights scouring Pinterest, planning the menu, gluing storylines to Popsicle sticks, and transforming our small space into a veritable garden. And the party, by all accounts, was a success. Not that my baby girl will remember it, but still. I will.

So when I placed the platter of leftover caterpillar-shaped cake on the kitchen counter, I felt entitled to an extra piece. *I deserve this*, I told myself, and wolfed down the sugary concoction. And then I had another piece. And another. And, well, there was only one more piece left in the row now, so I might as well finish it off.

At that moment, I heard the door open as my brother brought in an armful of decorations to drop off on the kitchen table. I felt myself turning three shades of red as I gulped down the mouthful of cake and quickly deposited the fork in the sink, hoping he wouldn't notice.

I walked out with him to finish cleaning up the party scene, but soon found myself in the kitchen again. I stole another few bites of cake, this time large heaping forkfuls, as if fewer bites (no matter how big) meant fewer calories.

As we continued to strip our garage of green and purple decorations, I repeatedly found my way to the kitchen when no one was looking, ingesting one huge bite of cake after another. I looked down at the diminished caterpillar, and even as I shoved another forkful of cake in my mouth, I wondered at my behavior.

I certainly wasn't hungry—I had long ago passed the point of feeling full.

And I wasn't unhappy—everyone had been lovely.

And I didn't really want more cake—truth be told, I was starting to feel a bit sick to my stomach. But even as I marveled at my lack of self-control, I kept eating.

I gravitated toward that cake like a moth toward a flame. No amount of logic or willpower could make me stop, and by the end of the night, I had eaten a quarter sheet of chocolate-vanilla birthday cake.

What just happened? I wondered, eying the demolished cake. Sure, I had binged before, but never to this extent. That night marked a new low in my food journey, and I felt disgusted with myself.

After I crashed from my sugar high, I made the drastic decision to undergo the Whole30 challenge. I resolved to eliminate all dairy, wheat, and sugar from my diet for thirty days. It sounded impossible, but I knew I needed a strict diet to get back on track. So the next day I made eggs for breakfast and headed out the door to work. I ate salad for lunch (sans dressing) and skipped the bread bowl at dinner. Other than wondering what to eat and constantly feeling unsatisfied, those first few days weren't too bad.

But then Day 4 came, and I felt like a truck hit me. I was cranky, irritable, lightheaded, and couldn't focus to save my life. My coworkers immediately noticed the change in me, and several expressed concern. I laughed it off as sugar withdrawal, but as the day went on, I hardly recognized myself. I wanted to punch someone in the face just for talking to me, and I thought the nice lady who had brought brownies to share deserved a three-day suspension.

One of my coworkers asked me why I thought I was behaving so oddly. I gave him the sugar withdrawal line, and he said, "Okay, maybe. But this isn't you. This is like Dr. Jekyll and Mr. Hyde. You're exactly opposite the person I know. Why is sugar, or rather, the lack of sugar, doing this to you?"

His words settled deep in the pit of my stomach. He was right. Though I had shrugged off my behavior as inconsequential, a simple symptom that would soon be over, the fact that I had crashed so hard was no laughing matter. I was behaving like a drug addict in rehab, and the similarities made me realize that sugar had a stronger hold on me than I thought. I didn't like the person I was when I was off sugar.

The symptoms continued for another three days, and they got worse before they got better. I even considered calling off work the next day because I didn't want to say or do something that I would later regret, like issuing that suspension over the yummy brownies that still haunted my dreams. I marveled at the change in me, and my husband, Flaviu, even suggested that this "crazy experiment" wasn't worth it.

"Just have a piece of chocolate cake," he suggested, good-naturedly. "I want my wife back."

But competitive person that I am, I pushed through, and on Day 8 I woke up to find my cravings had disappeared. I felt like I had just survived a monsoon in the middle of the ocean, and the waters had suddenly become calm as the sun poked through the clouds. I stopped craving food, and the platter of cookies that sat next to me at work that day didn't faze me in the least. I even smiled at the thoughtful person who brought them in.

That whole week I marveled at the transformation. Gradually, I stopped feeling hungry; in fact, I stopped having an appetite at all. This scared me, but for once I was free of the sugar monster perched on my shoulders, and I was okay with that. I felt a renewed sense of energy as my body went into ketosis, burning high amounts of stored fat to survive.

As I drove home from work one day, I realized that this is what it feels like to be free from food addiction, to finally control what and how I eat. This utter indifference toward food was new to me, and I felt empowered. I began skipping meals, and the lack of hunger encouraged me to keep cutting food out. My body changed also, and I liked the feel of my slender tummy and how my jeans began fitting more loosely every week. The power was intoxicating.

But alarm bells were also sounding. I recognized the beginning signs of an eating disorder and my husband and mom expressed concern as well. After the thirty days were over, I abandoned the diet for fear of slipping into a more dangerous eating pattern. But with no plan of reentry into the large world of food, I soon slipped into my old habits of eating everything I desired—and more.

My weight began to pile back on, and I was back on the food addiction roller coaster, binge-eating, gaining weight, then dieting a few weeks, only to slip into another binge and throw the whole plan out the window, gorging on food some more. As high as my victory felt during the thirty-day challenge, the crash of the following weeks was lower still.

I began researching the world of food disorders and diets. I wanted to get off the diet roller coaster, and as my little baby turned into a toddler, I wanted to model for her a healthy relationship with food. I didn't want her to inherit my food struggles.

Our problem is not really what we eat. It's why we seek fullness in something that will never satisfy.

In the months that followed, without even realizing the shift, I had gone from food addiction to food fixation: I became obsessed with thoughts and longings for food. At times I would daydream about living a healthy life, filled with green smoothies, quinoa bowls, kale salads, and three-mile runs. And just a few minutes later I would see a brownie-cheesecake-chocolate-chip-cookie concoction on Pinterest and immediately abandon my best intentions as I started toward the kitchen.

I spent hours each day scouring forums and scanning websites, reading books and pinning graphics, collecting recipes and noting best practices. Conversations centered around the diet tips and tricks my friends and I had tried that worked (and didn't), and it soon became apparent that many of them were as obsessed as I was to solve our "food problem."

I knew I wanted to eat real foods, in as close to their original state as possible. I wanted a sustainable approach that led to lots of energy and a healthy weight. And I wanted to feel trim and in control of my food choices instead of controlled by them. I read about paleo, low-carb, low-glycemic, and even several "biblical" diets. But no matter how many diets I looked at, none of them held an answer. I knew what and how to eat, but when I faced my favorite comfort foods, I lost all willpower to eat healthfully.

Food had ungodly control over me, and no amount of rules was going to change that.

Little did I know that I'd find the solution not in a diet but in the Word of God. The answer to food fixation does not lie in the $500 billion global diet industry but in our own laps.

We can't solve a spiritual problem with a physical solution. No matter whether we're eating healthfully or bingeing on comfort foods, we will not find the satisfaction we seek until we realize our cravings are meant to point us to God. God created us with hunger and cravings so that, by any means necessary, we will turn to Him.

This is not a diet book and it's not a healthy eating plan. You won't find recipes or swap-out recommendations here. Because, at the core, our problem is not really *what* we eat. It's *why* we seek fullness in something that will never satisfy. We don't need another diet; we need the sanctification that comes by the power of the Spirit. That's the only solution that leads to lasting change and creates in us the transformation that pleases God.

In the chapters that follow, you will discover the joy of living free from food fixation so you can experience deeper satisfaction in Christ, gain a renewed sense of purpose, and yes, enjoy good food.

This book is about discovering a deep satisfaction in Jesus that outlasts the richest meals, and finding that, in God, our stomachs and our souls can be full indeed.

Digest the truth
(for individual or group response)

1. Have you ever felt out of control when it comes to food? What happened? How did you feel afterwards? In what ways did that situation influence your current posture toward food?

2. How much pain does your food fixation cause you emotionally, physically, mentally, spiritually, relationally? What costs have you faced as you've wrestled with this issue in the past?

3. What types of diets have you tried? What food philosophies scare you or put you off? Do you prefer an eating plan that tells you exactly what to eat at each meal, or do you prefer general guidelines with flexibility?

4. What would it mean to you to finally conquer your food struggle? What would your life look like?

Bonus Online Content
Watch Asheritah share the reason she wrote this book, and download a prayer journal to record your reflections and progress at http://www.thefull.life/reading-journal.

Part One

Getting Real
about Our
Food Problem

1

Know That Calories Aren't the Enemy

Early in my food journey, I had resigned myself to a lifetime of yo-yo diets, guilt, deprivation, shame, and defeat.

"I guess this is my thorn in the flesh." I sighed as I approached the dessert table at a baby shower.

I envied the women around me who apparently had high metabolisms because they ate more than I did and still looked like skinny teenagers. But even more I envied those who weren't swayed by cravings. They would look at the dessert offerings, see nothing they wanted, and walk away without a second thought.

I, on the other hand, felt a magnetic pull toward decadent sweets whether I wanted them or not because, well, *hello, sugar rush!* It was as if another person inhabited my body for those five to ten minutes it would take me to wolf down a plate loaded with treats—a person who lacked self-control, long-term vision, and common sense. And glancing around the room at my friends, I knew I wasn't the only one having this out-of-body experience. Many of them looked just as ashamed and disappointed as I felt.

A week later, while sitting across from one of those women unfazed by a chocolate éclair, I confessed to her my struggle with food. And her response shocked me.

"Asheritah," she began, taking my hands in hers and gazing deeply into my eyes to the very bottom of my soul, right there in the middle of the coffee shop, "it doesn't have to be this way. You don't have to struggle for the rest of your life. Jesus can set you free from your struggle with food. He has for me."

I was shocked.

It had never occurred to me that my struggle with food was something that could be broken by Jesus. I never thought this was a spiritual issue. Sure, I had prayed before that God would help me lose the baby weight or that He'd forgive me for blowing my healthy eating plan yet again, but I had never asked Him to break the chains of my fixation and set me free.

My friend's words echoed in my mind during the days that followed. I realized that my problem wasn't the ten pounds I'd lose and gain year after year. The real problem was that the enemy had gained a corner of my life—my eating—and was using it to taunt me, distract me, and keep me living in bondage.

I saw that he had lured me with cookies and chips, promising immediate gratification to keep me from running to my Father. He was using my cravings to keep me chained to the desires of my flesh so I wouldn't let the Spirit take complete control of me.

I was mad at the enemy, broken over my ignorance, and yet hopeful as I clung to Jesus' promise to set me free.

And, friends, as I will share with you throughout this book, He *has* set me free, not all at once but through a gradual awakening to His surpassing sweetness. No comfort food can match the comfort I've found in Jesus.

Not Just a "Fat Girl" Problem

I've always been, as one writer put it, on the round side of average. Sometimes, especially in the winter, I'm on the fluffier end of that spectrum, while other times I'm on the more slender end. I enjoy good food, but I'm not the type of person most would peg as someone who has an eating problem.

In fact, it took that disastrous chocolate cake episode to make me acknowledge that I indeed did have an eating problem, and I needed to get help. In the months that followed, I began to open up to my close friends, sharing with them that I thought I was addicted to food.

Too many adults in the United States are trapped in a cycle of dieting, binge eating, and guilt tripping, only to gain back more weight than they lost. But it's not just overweight people who may struggle with an inordinate preoccupation with thoughts and longings for food. Whether it's skinny lattes, French fries, or Oreos, many Christian women feel powerless over their food fixation.

To my surprise, nearly every woman I talked with confessed that she, too, felt she had a food addiction, even when she knew she would suffer negative consequences, whether snugger jeans, bellyaches, migraines, or even health complications down the road. Rather than experience shame and condemnation as I had expected, there was a sense of camaraderie, a shared suffering that many of us felt but few of us spoke of honestly.

Even some of my skinny friends confessed that all day they thought about food. Some of them counted calories with every bite and performed mental gymnastics in determining whether or not they could have a bite of dessert. Others were converts of a popular eating program that was almost religious in its restrictions and influence, but they were constantly extolling the virtues of the newest power food.

Still others were committed to eating a healthy diet, locally sourced and certified organic, but they obsessed over the nutrients and origin of every ingredient they purchased to the point that a simple shopping trip drained them of all energy. Food fixation seemed to equally affect women of all ages, sizes, and religions; brownie lovers and kale lovers alike; underweight and obese; my Christian friends and I just as desperate in this issue as the atheist next door.

Food fixation is oppressive, enslaving us with thoughts and habits that torment and overpower us: "'What will I eat next? How much do I weigh today? What do others think of me? Why can't I get free of this? Why can't I be like others?' The same questions fill our thoughts over and over as we agonize day after day, looking for answers.'"

What Is Food Fixation, Anyway?

You might not have heard of the term *food fixation* before, but I'm sure you've heard of its close cousin—*gluttony.*

I don't know what you picture when you hear the word *glutton,* but for me it conjures images of stout men in a dark, eighteenth-century inn, sitting at a long wooden table, mugs sloshing with beer while chomping into a chicken thigh and singing raunchy lyrics. I guess it's just not a word I've connected with personally before, but it's one that appears in the Bible several times, so it helps to pay attention to it.

Let's define food fixation as "the inordinate preoccupation with thoughts and longings for food."

Biblically, the word *glutton* means a person who is debased and excessive in his or her eating habits. But it's more than just overeating—in its association with drunkenness in Scripture, it describes a life given to excess.[2] So while we tend to consider gluttony an action, we need to focus on the internal process that happens before, during, and after a gluttonous incident. For our purposes, let's define food fixation as *the inordinate preoccupation with thoughts and longings for food.*

Though we might not like to think of that extra serving of mac and cheese as a sin, God looks at the heart, and when we are controlled by something other than the Spirit of God, that is sin. Peter puts it this way in his letter to first-century believers: "People are slaves to whatever has mastered them" (2 Peter 2:19). Notice that the issue is not enjoying good food. After all, God is the one who created both our taste buds and the delicious ingredients used to make creative and delectable concoctions. The sin lies in seeking satisfaction in a sugar rush or endorphin high—that is, something other than God.

Think about it: whether we're controlled by pride, greed, alcohol, lust, or gluttony, the sin is not first in the action but rather in the influence; what needs to be rooted out is whatever controls us in our hearts, and only then will our outer actions change. In other words, until we deal with the heart issue of seeking fullness in food instead of God, our eating habits will never change.

As one writer explains, "Eating habits become sinful when the habitual practice of them places us in bondage again—a bondage to sin from which Christ died to free us."[3] This bondage may be physical, like a sugar addiction, or it may be mental, such as investing excessive mental energy into planning healthy meals. We need to plead with the Spirit to reveal to us and convict us of any sin in our lives, including gluttony, idolatry, addiction, and anything else.

When we eat and eat and eat, unaware of what's going into our mouths, unable to taste, enjoy, or relish the food but just stuffing down one mouthful after another until it makes us sick—that's being enslaved to our appetites.

We can also allow pride to drive even commendable eating habits because again, the problem is in those root issues of the heart more than in our external actions. For example, scores of women today are trapped by their "healthy eating" plan. This type of gluttony may not be self-evident, because it's common to keep such tight control of what and how much is eaten; but it is precisely in the need to control every bite that this type of gluttony is also an enslavement to food and appetites.

When one insists on eating only organic, only natural, only homemade, only whatever, to the exasperation of friends and family and hostesses, that woman is controlled by her food choices, not vice versa. This, too, is a form of food fixation.

So while the Bible does not speak of *food fixation* specifically, we will soon see that it has much to say about its various manifestations in our lives.

Answer the Invitation

After a hard day of work, a bowl of ice cream seems to be the perfect answer to my problems—for about five minutes. After the sugar rush wears off, I'm left feeling just as tired, worn out, and empty as before, but now there's guilt and disillusionment piled on top! Might as well have another bowl, right?

The truth is I only compound my misery when I take my brokenness to the fridge. Food cannot fix anything—God is the only one who can satisfy us because He created us to find our satisfaction in Him.

Our journey from food fixation to lasting fullness begins with an invitation issued thousands of years ago:

> Come, all you who are thirsty, come to the waters; and you who have no money, come, buy and eat! Come, buy wine and milk without money and without cost. Why spend money on what is not bread, and your labor on what does not satisfy? Listen, listen to me, and eat what is good, and your soul will delight in the richest of fare. (Isaiah 55:1–2)

In the context of this passage, the nation of Israel had spent her time and energy on idols that promised to fill the void but left the people empty and broken. Yet God responded not with disappointment, anger, or vengeance but with a loving invitation. He longed for the Israelites to return to Him, just as He longs for us to return and find true satisfaction in Him.

How interesting that God would use food imagery to communicate His desire that we find comfort and satisfaction in Him alone. And not just any food—He invites His people to feast on a veritable banquet: wine and milk—symbols of abundance, enjoyment, and nourishment.

God isn't a cosmic killjoy. In fact, delicious food and working taste buds were His idea in the first place. He's not out to ruin our pleasure in good food. Rather, He wants us to abandon our self-constructed salvation projects and turn to Him instead, urging us to listen to Him and "eat" and find delight in the best this world has to offer: God Himself.

But anyone who has ever tried to change her eating habits will readily attest that it's not easy. Changing behaviors we've spent years practicing takes more than a freshly printed eating plan and a fridge full of fruits and veggies. No, overcoming food fixation will require more than we've ever imagined, and it will reward us with more than we ever dreamed possible.

What is at stake is not just the extra pounds we've accumulated year by year. It's not our health or our vitality or our energy levels. It's not fitting into that swimsuit in time for our summer vacation or finally feeling comfortable in our skin. What's at stake is much more valuable than that, and it's of eternal significance. This is a battle of epic proportions. Food will never satisfy us because it was never meant to. God created food for many reasons, but providing emotional comfort was never one of them.

———

Looking to the Israelites back then and to us now with affection, God lovingly uses imagery He knows we will relate to—food—as a metaphor for the spiritual refreshment He wants us to discover in Him. And the life He offers isn't merely survival—that would just be bread and water. No, He offers us an abundance of spiritual blessings in Christ Jesus, all we could ever want and more!

Quite simply, we face a choice: we can continue to stuff ourselves with food, hoping that one more meal will fill us, or we can recognize that we were never made to live on food alone. Our souls were created to crave God, and as St. Augustine confessed so long ago, "Our hearts are restless until they find rest in You."

If you're ready to get off the hamster wheel of diets and try-harder plans, I invite you to join me at the table of God's presence. He is the only one who can satisfy, and He's happy to do so.

Find Real Comfort and Satisfaction

We all seek comfort and satisfaction in one place or another. Some of us turn to relationships, TV shows, shopping, or alcohol. Others of us turn to food. In and of themselves, none of these things are bad, but each of these good gifts can quickly become idols, taking on importance and influence that should only belong to God.

At its core, food fixation is an issue of idolatry, just like any other addiction, because it doesn't just affect our health, our relationships, and our lives, but it hinders our relationship with God.

For many of us, it's easier to ignore our food struggles than admit we have a problem. We tell ourselves, "Oh, it's just an extra bite," or "I'm not hurting anyone," as we plunge into the sleeve of cookies. Year after year, diet after diet, we continue to delude ourselves. We're not sure what we will find if we allow God to shine His light of truth into our hearts. We're afraid we won't like what we see, that we won't have the strength to face the years of hurt we've stuffed down inside, that God will call us to a yoke that is too heavy for us to bear.

If the idea of food as an idol seems strange to you, ask yourself if any of these statements are true of you:[4]

> I could never give up my favorite food.
>
> I spend more time and energy thinking about food than I do growing in my relationship with Christ.
>
> I find more delight and happiness in food than in my relationship with Christ.

If you answered yes to any of the statements above, chances are you're turning to food as an idol, seeking comfort in a fleeting bite rather than in God.

What's your favorite food? The one you eat to forget about a bad day at work or to celebrate a big accomplishment? Picture yourself sitting down with a generous serving. Imagine how great it tastes, how it hits the spot, how even the thought of indulging in it brings anticipation and excitement. Whether it's homemade lasagna, luscious apple pie, avocado slathered on toast, or an ice-cold cola, these foods provide only temporary satisfaction. Shortly after we've left the table, we've already forgotten the deliciousness of the meal as the day's problems and worries invade our mind.

These comfort foods provide us a glimmer of the satisfaction God wants to offer us if we let Him. And if anyone knew what it was like to need lasting comfort and satisfaction, it was the apostle Paul. After becoming the leading missionary to the Gentiles, Paul experienced extreme persecution, pain, and suffering. But in the midst of it all, he was filled to the measure with the comfort of God.

Take a look at this beautiful passage: "Praise be to the God and Father of our Lord Jesus Christ, the Father of compassion and the God of all comfort, who comforts us in all our troubles, so that we can comfort those in any trouble with the comfort we ourselves receive from God" (2 Corinthians 1:3–4).

The word "comfort" appears four times in just these two verses. Paul says that the God of *comfort comforts* us so that we may *comfort* others with the *comfort* we've received from God. Paul writes from personal experience, as God poured His comfort into Paul's heart.

In *Looking for Lovely,* Annie Downs describes the night she discovered she had a food problem. Sitting on the couch, eating popcorn and watching a reality TV show featuring a cocaine addict, Annie came face to face with the gravity of her food struggle:

> I had an addiction. For over twenty years I had taken
> all the pain and hurt and pushed it straight down my
> throat. For as much as I read the Bible, sat in Sunday

school, and made the church my second home, I wish I'd understood, "His ears are open for their cries for help" (Ps. 34:15). Instead of feeling any of the suffering, instead of pressing through the pain and taking it to God, trusting that He heard me, I escaped to anywhere that would feed me, and I stuffed my emotions down by covering them in layers of food. What if I had found cocaine instead of candy? What if I had drunk beer instead of a milkshake? . . . I have the same propensity as any other addict; it's just my drug of choice is food.[5]

What a sobering thought, that many of us turn to food as an alcoholic turns to brandy, or a drug addict turns to heroin. Somehow, we can trick ourselves into thinking our food fixation isn't that big of a deal when we're simply munching on a cookie. But at the heart of the issue, we're all doing the same thing. Wouldn't you rather experience the fullness of God's comfort than the emptiness of a sugar-induced guilt trip the next time you reach for the Oreos?

Food Is Not the Enemy

A National Health and Nutrition Examination Survey found that over 60 percent of women in the United States are overweight and 40 percent of women are obese.[6] These numbers are alarming, especially since obesity is linked to high blood pressure, heart disease, and many other illnesses. And of course, the food we eat affects our health and our weight; most of us have been on at least one diet in an effort to curb our growing waistlines, even while our culture idolizes skinny bodies.

So we've come to hate our appearance, fear our appetites, and view food as the enemy.

But food is not the enemy. Food is a good gift from a good God given to direct our hearts in worship to the Father. In fact, Jesus enjoyed food while He lived on this earth; He knew both how to feast and to fast. Here are just a few of the scenes in which Jesus relates to food that we glimpse in the Bible:

> Jesus fasted forty days in the wilderness in preparation for His public ministry (Matthew 4:1–4).
>
> Jesus taught His disciples to not worry about food and drink because God will take care of them (Matthew 6:25–26).
>
> Jesus dined with tax collectors and sinners, while the Pharisees called Him a "glutton and a drunkard" (Matthew 11:19).
>
> Jesus gave instructions regarding who to invite to dinner parties (Luke 14:12–14).
>
> Jesus had compassion on the crowds who were following Him without enough food for dinner, so He miraculously provided food for all (Matthew 14:15–21).
>
> Jesus defended His disciples' lack of fasting during His lifetime, explaining that they will fast when He's gone (Mark 2:20).
>
> Jesus made careful preparations to eat the Passover meal with His disciples before the crucifixion (Luke 22:7–13).

Jesus chose bread and wine as symbols His followers would use to remember His sacrifice (Luke 22:14–20).

Jesus thanked God for meals and broke bread before and after His resurrection (Luke 24:28–31).

Jesus asked the disciples if they had food to eat after His resurrection (Luke 24:41–43).

Jesus made breakfast for His disciples after His resurrection (John 21:9–13).

Jesus used dinner parties and wedding banquets as pictures of the future kingdom of God (Matthew 22:2; Luke 14:16–24).

What do these vignettes tell us about the way Jesus related to food? He didn't ignore His appetite, but He wasn't controlled by it either. He was able to both fast and feast, and He often gathered people around the table to fellowship at a deeper level. We could spend an entire chapter unpacking each of these passages and learning so much more just from Jesus' example in His relationship with food. But the overarching theme here is that Jesus ate food while on earth and also indicated that food would be a reality in the coming kingdom of God. Food is not a bad thing, but food fixation can easily become a stronghold in our lives if we're not careful.

A Spiritual Battle

When God created us, He purposefully placed our souls and spirits inside bodies. He set in place the digestive system to process food and convert it into energy, and then He developed our brain chemistry to link foods to emotions and memories. Finally, He used food to illustrate truths about our spirits that we could not fathom otherwise. In so many ways, food is a delectable gift given to us by a Father who delights in us.

But like any good gift, our appetites have been targeted by the enemy in an effort to thwart God's plan. It's become common to blame our national health crisis in America on food corporations and greedy executives. Obesity rates are through the roof; diabetes, heart disease, and cancer have become household guests that refuse to leave; and more than half of American adults depend on at least two daily medications.[7] Scientists have linked many of our illnesses to increased artificial ingredients in our diets, so our anger toward the food industry is justifiable. But it is misplaced.

Satan will use whatever tool he can to distract people from seeking satisfaction in God, and if money, sex, or power don't hold any sway over you, then French fries or skinny chocolate lattes just might.

Corporations are not our enemy. Behind the suits, the bank accounts, and the fake food lobbyists there stands a demonic force. I'm not being melodramatic here. Jesus Himself said that Satan and his minions have come to steal, kill, and destroy, and that's exactly what they're doing through the food and diet industries. But we have become so fixated with our protein shakes and diet plans that we fail to realize our food problem is, at its core, a spiritual one.

Paul affirms Jesus' words when he identifies our chief enemy as being Satan and the spiritual powers of darkness: "For our struggle is not against flesh and blood, but against the rulers, against the authorities, against the powers of this dark world and against the spiritual forces of evil in the heavenly realms" (Ephesians 6:12). Let's not be fooled into thinking that the health crisis facing us today is coincidental. Satan will use whatever tool he can to distract people from seeking satisfaction in God, and if money, sex, or power don't hold any sway over you, then French fries or skinny chocolate lattes just might. He doesn't care what our favorite drug is as long as it keeps us running away from God.

Friends, this battle we're fighting to break free from food fixation is not as simple as throwing out the junk food and skipping dessert. While those steps may be needed, we cannot ignore the role our souls and spirits play in this battle for satisfaction. This is a spiritual war that has seen many committed Christians captured as POWs or MIA. It is in brushing it off as no big deal or "just a few pounds a diet will take care of" that the enemy steals our will to fight. Why engage in warfare when I can kick back with another bowl of ice cream?

Why do we keep turning to food to give us something it was never made to do? If we've experienced the disappointment that follows a food binge, why do we continue to seek comfort in food?

The most obvious answer is our sinful nature; we will turn to anything and everything besides God to fill that void inside of us. Starting back in the garden of Eden, humans have been trying to be self-sufficient and autonomous but have failed miserably every time, because trying to mask our need for

God with food is like trying to pound a nail in the wall with an orange; we'll only end up frustrated and hurt.

But another reason we keep turning to food, even after it's failed us, is because for many of us, food fixation has become a stronghold in our lives.

Demolishing Strongholds

A stronghold is a place that has been fortified so as to protect it against attack. Imagine a fortress whose walls have been reinforced, fenced in with barbed wire, and surrounded by a moat. As an abstract concept, strongholds are anything that have a "strong hold" on us, making us feel powerless. Applied to our spiritual lives, a stronghold is any thought, fear, behavior, or belief that gains a place in our lives in bigger-than-life proportions. Anger, bitterness, unforgiveness are common ones. And food fixation can be a stronghold.

When this happens, food fixation steals our attention and our focus, making us feel controlled and mastered. As Beth Moore explains, "It consumes so much of our emotional and mental energy that abundant life is strangled—our callings remain largely unfulfilled and our believing lives are virtually ineffective," which is exactly what the enemy wants.[8]

For those of us who have identified the stronghold of food fixation, we can probably relate to that definition. Food fixation is a constant presence that taints every other aspect of our lives and leaves us feeling discouraged and hopeless.

And most of us have probably tried using the world's weapons to fight it: we've been on countless diets, read lots of books, tried low-fat recipes, bought fad miracle-foods, and spent an embarrassing number of hours dreaming of what life will be like once we're finally free from this struggle.

But that hasn't worked.

We're still struggling. And the reason we're struggling is because we're trying to fight a spiritual battle with worldly weapons. I don't mean to go all wonky on you here, but I firmly believe that the food struggles many of us face are part of Satan's master plan to keep us away from God. If you believe that Satan exists, then you better believe he and his minions are fighting as hard as they can to keep you looking for satisfaction in all the wrong places.

> There is an enemy and he is after something in your life and it is the truth. And I fear that we do not take [this] seriously enough.... If I were your enemy, I would make you numb and distract you from God's story. I would use technology, social media, Netflix, travel, food, wine, comfort. And I wouldn't tempt you with notably bad things or you would get suspicious. I would distract you with everyday comforts that slowly feed you a different story and make you forget God. Then you would dismiss the Spirit's leading in you, loving you and comforting you, then you would love comfort more than surrender, obedience, and the saving of souls.[9]

The truth is that there is an enemy and he's out to destroy us. And if he can't destroy us because we're eternally secure in the arms of God, then he will seek to debilitate us, rendering us useless for God's kingdom work here on earth. This is a real battle, and it's raging all around us even in this moment.

So let's put down the weapons of this world: the diets, the fads, the positive thinking, and take up God's weapons: prayer, the Word of God, and the Spirit of God.

The apostle Paul knew all about the realities of the spiritual world. If he were sitting down with us over a meal (try tilapia, flat bread, hummus, and pomegranates), I'm convinced he'd tell us we need to get more serious about spiritual warfare and eternity. Take a look at what he says about spiritual battles: "For though we live in the world, we do not wage war as the world does. The weapons we fight with are not the weapons of the world. On the contrary, they have divine power to demolish strongholds" (2 Corinthians 10:3–4).

Paul speaks into our struggle, reassuring us that victory can be ours, but it won't come by using the same weapons nonbelievers use. Overcoming food fixation isn't simply about making a few substitutions and exercising self-control. This battle is fought primarily in the spiritual realm, and the battlefield is our minds.

But before we start, I need to warn you that we have an unfair advantage: our weapons have divine power to demolish strongholds. *Divine power.* We don't need to feel pressured to win this battle because it's already won! What we're about to embark on is a journey of learning to rely on God's power to do for us what we can't on our own: annihilate the bigger-than-life struggle that has haunted us for so long. And He *delights* in fighting this battle for us because it brings us closer to Him.

Please don't misunderstand me: I'm not saying that if you simply follow a spiritual formula, all your health problems will disappear. That's not what Scripture tells us. What I *am* saying is that God created us as three-personed beings, with bodies, souls, and spirits, and we will experience victory in our food struggles when we recognize the spiritual component of this battle for satisfaction.

You won't find diet advice in this book, but that doesn't mean you should ignore common-sense nutritional and exercise advice. Find a healthy eating plan that works for you (body), and then delve into this book to learn how to transform your thoughts and feelings about food (soul), and satisfy your hunger for God in His presence (spirit). When we address all three components together, we will be wise to our enemy's plans and finally discover the fullness of life we've been searching for all along.

As we pick up these spiritual weapons and engage in the battle of our lives, we will experience God mightily working in us to break the power of anything that has a hold on us and command it to bend the knee to the authority of Jesus Christ. Overcoming food fixation will be a challenge. It will require full dedication, spiritual preparation, and divine intervention.

But we don't have to fight this battle for lasting satisfaction on our own. God Himself promises to empower us, strengthen us, change us, and carry us day by day, as our souls gradually awaken to the satisfying sweetness of His presence, transforming us into the likeness of His Son until we finally reach heaven.

Are you ready?

Digest the Truth

(*for individual or group response*)

1. What does the term *food fixation* mean to you? Do you think it's possible to become obsessive in think-

ing about food, eating, clipping recipes, talking about diets, food fads, etc.? Have you known someone who was overly fascinated with food, even if they weren't necessarily physically overweight? Have you experienced it? What was the result?

2. Why do you want to overcome food fixation? What's your primary motivation?

3. Do you believe food fixation is a spiritual battle? Why or why not? How does your response change your approach to losing weight, eating healthy, or whatever your food goal is?

4. What does your ideal relationship with food look like? Describe how you'd feel about it, how you would eat, what you would think, and how you would act in this ideal lifestyle. What's your goal on this journey?

5. What relationship do you notice in your own life between physical, mental, and spiritual fullness (or emptiness) and food fixation? What habits do you need to develop to live life to the full?

6. Which of the scenes in which Jesus relates to food struck you the most? What can we learn from each of those passages?

Bonus Online Content

Join the 10-day email challenge to receive extra devotionals and action points at http://www.thefull.life/challenge.

2

Dress for Success

I'm by nature a competitive person. This explains why I jumped at the thirty-day paleo challenge, why I completed a seven-day green smoothie challenge, and why my husband can get me to do anything by simply turning it into a game.

When I think of spiritual warfare, I tend to picture epic battle scenes from *Braveheart*, *Gladiator*, and the Lord of the Rings series. I think of massive armies colliding in valleys with clashing swords, sweat and blood flying everywhere, adrenaline pumping as one army overtakes the other.

So it surprised me to discover that God doesn't call us to charge into battle and chase away the enemy. Our battle is not one massive invasion of the domain of darkness but rather individual victory in hand-to-hand combat, time after time after time.

This battle is not won in one fell swoop; it is won incrementally, each time we stand firm in God's truth and cling to Him for comfort. It's telling that Paul, in the classic passage on spiritual warfare, charges his readers to simply stand firm: "Finally, be strong in the Lord and in his mighty power. Put on the full armor of God, so that you can stand against the devil's schemes" (Ephesians 6:10–11).

Four times in Ephesians 6:10–14 Paul writes that we are to stand, and the same is true in our battle with food. Each time we choose God instead of food, our stronghold loses a bit of its power over us. Victory over our enemy takes time, as we repeatedly choose God over anything else that promises to satisfy.

Scientists are now finding that food addiction acts on the brain in ways similar to other chemical addictions: when excess sugar is ingested, it stimulates the brain "in such a way that it is easy to get hooked and tough to break free, even if you find yourself gaining weight or lapsing into health problems." And this addictive quality isn't just limited to sugar; it can be triggered by chocolate, cheese, meat, caffeine, and other foods.[1]

Additionally, food addiction suppresses the release of serotonin (the chemical in our brain that indicates fullness) and stimulates beta-endorphins, the chemicals that communicate pleasure and well-being.[2] Like with many other addictions though, these receptors require higher and higher doses to deliver the same level of satisfaction.

Starving the brain receptors of the stimulants initially leads to withdrawal symptoms such as headaches, chills, lightheadedness, and fever but will give way to detoxification, and in time allow you to overcome the addiction.[3] In other words, repeatedly choosing God over food will eventually help our brains return to healthy nonaddictive functioning, making the journey easier. But it gets harder before it gets easier.

The Holy Spirit is involved every step of the way, training us to know the difference between righteous and unrighteous eating, empowering us to stop carrying out the desire of the flesh that we exhibit with our eating (Romans 8:13); teaching us how to eat in a way that is pleasing to Him (John 16:13); changing us through the truth (2 Thessalonians 2:13). As we put off our old self and put on the new, the Holy Spirit will transform our thinking (see Ephesians 4:22–24).

We cannot rely on our own willpower to overcome food fixation, because we'll eventually reach its limit. When we get weary, our mind, will, and emotions want to do what's easy,

We must remember that we stand not in our own power but in the mighty power of God.

even if that results in our destruction. But the Holy Spirit of God leads us to victory, and we're to follow His lead in our lives: "Let the Holy Spirit guide your lives. Then you won't be doing what your sinful nature craves" (Galatians 5:16 NLT).

While we need willpower and discipline to create healthy habits, those things alone will only take us so far (as anyone who's started a diet only to fail will tell you). Instead of relying on our own willpower, let us beg God for a fresh outpouring of His Holy Spirit in our lives. "'Not by might nor by power, but by my Spirit' says the Lord Almighty" (Zechariah 4:6). His Holy Spirit infuses our willpower with His supernatural resources, energizing us to cross the finish line. This way, we don't get credit for our success—all glory goes to God. He is the one who helps us stand firm in our battle for finding satisfaction in God alone.

We learn to stand firm in several ways:

Running to God instead of food

Whenever I'm hankering for something sweet, I can recognize the urge as my brain telling me it wants immediate gratification. When I instead take a moment to pray about what's on my mind, I interrupt that addictive habit and form a new habit, one that provides infinitely more satisfying comfort in God.

Choosing healthy meal options

I discovered that I crave the foods I eat.[4] If I binge on potato chips, sweet rolls, and soda, I'll crave those foods more strongly. But if I stay away from the artificial stuff and fill my plate with a rainbow of foods from God's green earth, I'm reinforcing my brain's God-given reward system to recognize that healthy foods are good for me, and that's what I'll begin craving instead.

Filling our minds with truth

Every time I'm ambushed by lies (like "I deserve this" or "I've got to have this") and fight them with truth, I'm reinforcing the supremacy of God's Word over the enemy's lies. The more often I assert truth, the more naturally it will come to mind.

We must remember that we stand not in our own power but in the mighty power of God. If you're reading this book, you're probably desperate for victory because you've tried diets and exercise programs, and they haven't worked. Those things alone will help you lose ten or fifteen pounds, but soon enough you'll have slipped off the plan and packed on the pounds. Again.

This cycle of yo-yo dieting is familiar to many and is precisely the reason we can't overcome food addiction on our own. We need God. And the wonderful news is that He's more than happy to help. In fact, He's given us everything we need to be successful.

Wise to the Enemy's Plans

In our journey toward learning to find satisfaction in God alone, we have an enemy whose goal is to use any means necessary to destroy us. Jesus said as much: "The thief comes only to steal and kill and destroy; I have come that they may have life, and have it to the full" (John 10:10).

For many of us, the enemy's preferred bait is food.

He steals our peace through consuming thoughts of food.

He steals our victory by luring us back into temptation.

He steals our joy by drawing us away from God, the only one who satisfies.

He also kills with food. Quite literally, the food we're putting into our bodies can cause diabetes, heart disease, cancer, and obesity.

But Satan also seeks to kill us spiritually, keeping us in spiritual darkness, blind to the life-giving elixir found only in Jesus Christ. Our enemy wants us to eat Twinkies after a stressful day instead of praying. He wants to wreck our testimony as lights in the darkness, causing us to eat and diet desperately just like the world does.

He is a roaring lion, seeking to steal, kill, and destroy. But we don't face him alone. Look at the second part of the verse: "I have come that they may have life, and have it to the full."

As you look back on your history of dieting, do you see patterns of life or death? Joy or sorrow? Celebration or desperation?

Jesus, our Good Shepherd, laid down His life so we could have abundant life, which includes experiencing victory and freedom in our eating. He endured what the enemy had planned for us: His glory was stolen, His life was snuffed out, and His ministry was destroyed.

Or so it seemed.

For a few dark days, the earth trembled and hell celebrated as the Son of God endured what each of us deserved. But hell's festivities were cut short by the resurrection of Jesus Christ, declaring His ultimate victory over sin, death, and destruction.

Satan has no power over us because Jesus has overcome! He is the resurrection and the life, and He offers us life abundantly.

As we understand who the enemy is and what he's after, we fight not with fear but with courage because Jesus has already overcome him.

Equipped for Battle

We have weapons at our disposal, as Paul explains:

Therefore, put on the full armor of God, so that when the day of evil comes, you may be able to stand your ground, and after you have done everything, to stand. Stand firm then, with the *belt of truth* buckled around your waist, with the *breastplate of righteousness* in place, and with your *feet fitted* with the readiness that

49

comes from the gospel of peace. In addition to all this, take up the *shield of faith*, with which you can extinguish all the flaming arrows of the evil one. Take the *helmet of salvation* and the *sword of the Spirit*, which is the word of God. And *pray* in the Spirit on all occasions with all kinds of prayers and requests. With this in mind, be alert and always keep on praying for all the Lord's people. (Ephesians 6:13–18)

Belt of Truth

The first item in our warfare wardrobe is the belt of truth. In ancient times, when a man prepared for battle, he'd tie up his loose, flowy robe and tuck it into his belt.[5] The belt held his outfit together; without it he would have tripped all over the place.

As we make food choices, we need to bring all our thoughts, emotions, hopes, and dreams and tuck them into the belt of truth, carefully examining which of them line up with God's Word and which should be discarded, as we'll discuss in the next chapter.

Breastplate of Righteousness

Next is the breastplate of righteousness, the armor that covers our hearts and protects us from fatal blows. In this battle to overcome food addiction, we must remember that Jesus Christ is our righteousness; He is the one who took our sins on Himself and paid the penalty of death. His righteousness is transferred to us and covers us, protecting us for all eternity.

We are safe and secure no matter what happens. We fight not to secure our righteousness before God but because of the righteousness that is already ours in Christ Jesus. Our self-control before that plate of cookies does not make God love us any more or any less than He already does. We must also remember that when we're tempted to turn our healthy eating plan into a legalistic list of dos and don'ts. Our healthy eating doesn't earn God's favor: Jesus already did that for us.

Sandals of Peace

We then slip on our footgear, the protective supportive equipment that is the gospel of peace. While this may refer to an eagerness to evangelize and witness to others about Jesus Christ, it may also be seen as the assurance that the battle is already won. The gospel of peace refers to the finished work of Jesus Christ to reconcile (make peace between) man and God. On the cross, Jesus declared, "It is finished," eliminating any need for human effort, good works, or the pressure to prove anything to God.

We stand ready to fight our food fixation because we have nothing to prove and everything to gain. We live at peace with God (John 14:27); as we invite Him into this area of our lives, we ask Him to flood us with His peace that transcends all understanding (Philippians 4:7). Because of Jesus Christ, I can live out the good news that God has already won the battle, and I need only to walk in His victory.

Shield of Faith

Next is our shield of faith. With it we protect ourselves from the enemy's arrows of doubt and despair. Our faith rests not in our own self-discipline or our proven track record (because, let's face it, our past failures inspire doubt, not courage); our faith rests in Jesus.

Whenever I begin to doubt whether this journey will be different from all the diets I've tried before, I stand firm in my faith in Jesus and His promises to satisfy me. God promises that if we seek Him with all our heart, we will find Him (Jeremiah 29:13), and that is our desire: to find satisfaction and comfort in God alone. God is faithful to His promises and He will never let us down. We can rely on Him.

Helmet of Salvation

We also put on the helmet of salvation, the part that protects our minds and reassures us that we are God's. Our salvation rests in Jesus Christ, not our performance.

No matter what victories or failures we experience, even if we slip up and make a mistake, we still belong to God and He will see us through.

Sword of the Spirit

The offensive weapon on this list is the sword of the Spirit, which is the Word of God. We wield this by studying His Word, memorizing it, and applying it to our lives. If you're not currently digging into the Bible, start now by looking up the texts referenced in this book.

When picking up this weapon, though, let us not forget that it is alive and active, brought to life by the Holy Spirit who indwells us and brings Jesus' words to mind. When we ask Him to lead and direct us, He will do so. The Word of God is not just writing on a page; it is the living, breathing presence of His Spirit in every believer. As we obey His promptings, His voice will become increasingly clear to us as the Word comes alive in our lives.

Prayer

Lastly, the whole armor is held together by prayer, our communication with God. Our default will be to try to fight this battle alone, but we must keep reminding ourselves that we depend on God for both comfort and strength. This is not just another diet or eating plan; this is a new way of living in the freedom of Jesus Christ. We need God to make that change in us as we stand firm in battle.

As we engage this battle day by day, there may be times when we feel like we don't even have the strength to form a prayer. Then God's Holy Spirit helps us by interceding on our behalf, interpreting our wordless groans into supplications before the Father (Romans 8:26–27). And the best part is He is able to pray for exactly what we need in each exact moment, because He knows both our struggle and God's thoughts toward us. We are not alone in this battle; the Holy Spirit of God is praying for us every step of the way.

As I'm tempted to choose the chips rather than the carrot sticks, I pray that God will give me wisdom, discernment, and strength. As I'm wandering through the house because I want to hit the secret chocolate stash, I pray that God will satisfy me with Himself. Prayer is essential to a believer's victory over food addiction. And God will always see us through.

Choosing Life . . . One Bite at a Time

God knows we have a tendency to turn away from Him with alarming velocity. As soon as I experience a bit of freedom from my cravings, I'm tempted to ditch God and forge my own path. I stop listening to the Spirit and just replicate what worked in the past. I begin to believe that I've won these victories all on my own. And then, inevitably, I relapse into my old eating habits.

We are called to choose life by loving God above all else.

This journey to overcome food fixation is not just about fitting into smaller jeans or figuring out clean eating. God's greatest desire isn't just to kick our sin to the curb; what He really wants is to draw us closer to His heart.

Look what Moses says: "Now choose life, so that you and your children may live and that you may *love* the Lord your God, *listen* to his voice, and *hold fast* to him. For the Lord is your life" (Deuteronomy 30:19–20).

We are called to choose life by loving God above all else, listening to His voice instead of the enemy's lies, and holding fast to Him for the rest of our lives. And we'll break down what that looks like throughout this book.

This food journey is simply a medium for Him to accomplish a greater work in our lives. What the enemy intended to destroy us, God will use for our good and His glory. Look at the next season of your life as an opportunity to allow God to do anything and everything to strip you of self-reliance and to knit your heart to His.

Ask Him to turn your shame and despair into worship and praise. Ask Him to use your lifelong struggle with food and the victories you'll experience to point other people to Jesus as well. View this as the beginning of a beautiful relationship, one that will grow deeper and more intimate the closer you grow to Him.

Like the Israelites, we must choose between life and death.

And when we choose life, we choose so much more than a temporary fix for our problem. We choose God Himself, for He is our life.

Digest the Truth

(for individual or group response)

1. Does it make sense to you that we need to put on spiritual armor when engaging in the battle to overcome food fascination? Explain. Have you ever consciously applied these principles to your efforts to right your relationship to food? If so, how? What can you do to prepare yourself for battle?

2. How can shame keep us from experiencing the full life God intends for us? When have you experienced shame about your appetite or body in your own life?

3. Do you believe that God is interested in your food fixation struggle? How does He manifest His interest?

4. Reflect on the past forty-eight hours. In what ways had God offered you escapes from temptation and strength to overcome? Did you obey or disobey? What were the consequences of your actions? How can you learn from that experience so you experience victory next time?

5. What is God calling you to change in your approach to food and fullness? Are you willing to commit yourself to the new life God offers you and give Him control of your eating? What might change if you do? What specific action will you take today to begin this journey of finding satisfaction in Jesus?

Bonus Online Content

Download "The Armor of God" printable at http://www.thefull.life/armor.

Laura's Story

When I was a teenager, my family moved from Romania to the United States; as I adopted the American lifestyle, the extra pounds began creeping on. I didn't think much of it until random women from church started commenting on my weight. Suddenly, losing weight began to consume me. It almost became an obsession—I tried all these diets, willing to do anything to lose the weight. But nothing seemed to work.

One day it hit me that my weight wasn't just a physical problem—it was a spiritual problem. I was running to food for comfort, and although I realized I couldn't change on my own, I didn't want to trouble God with this little thing when people were really hurting in the world. But then I realized we need to pray about everything, and God cares about the smallest details.

So I cried out to God, "Lord, You have to set me free because I can't go on like this." I prayed that same prayer for almost two years before I realized I had lost twenty-five pounds without even trying. I stopped thinking about food and instead focused on finding satisfaction in God, and He changed me. To this day, I still eat everything my friends do, but just eat less; I'm no longer obsessed with food or my looks, and I've learned to pray about everything.

3

Choose Truth
Over Lies

We sat around the kitchen table, taking turns sharing lies we believe and inviting each other to speak truth into our lives.

I was uncomfortable.

I had learned to trust these women and appreciated their encouragement every time I opened my soul. But sharing the most vulnerable parts of us is never easy, no matter how many times we take deep breaths and speak those first few shaky words. It's embarrassing to confess the thoughts we let rule our actions and the sins we commit when we think no one's looking.

But that day, as we went around the circle and spoke aloud those lies that had taken up residence in our minds, we began to see them for what they were: half-truths meant to enslave us.

Here are some of the lies I've believed about food. Perhaps you're familiar with them as well:

> I deserve that brownie! In fact, I've had such a stressful day, I should eat two.
>
> It's just a bag of chips. It's not a big deal, not like I'm smoking pot or something.
>
> If I don't eat that extra slice of pizza, who knows when I'll have another?
>
> This [insert favorite comfort food] is exactly what I need right now. It will make me feel better and make my problems go away.
>
> If God really loved me, He would set me free of this food addiction right now.
>
> This tastes so good! How can something that tastes so good be bad?
>
> God gave us taste buds, so there's no reason to hold back. I can dig in and eat all I want!
>
> I worked out hard this morning so I can eat whatever I want the rest of the day.

On and on those lies roll around in our minds and we get comfortable with them. They blend in with the chores to be done, the dry cleaning to pick up, and that new recipe to try this weekend. Those lies sneak through the back door and make themselves at home, and the longer they stay, the more we believe them.

It doesn't take much to defeat them. Really, five seconds is all it takes. But before we can look at the solution, we need to first understand where lies come from and why they're so insidious in the first place.

The Lie That Birthed All Others

Scripture tells us that our enemy, Satan, is the father of lies. In fact, Satan spoke the first lie in the history of the universe, and wouldn't you know it—it centered on food.

When God created the first man and woman, He placed them in the garden of Eden and gave them permission to eat from any tree except for one.

The first couple didn't lack variety or deliciousness in their diet. They freely ate their fill from the delicacies fashioned by God Himself. The fact that they couldn't eat from that one tree didn't bother them in the least because they had all they needed and more.

But then Satan slithered onto the scene in the form of a serpent. Notice that when he first started speaking to Eve, he tossed her a softball, something that would engage her in conversation and would allow him a little window of opportunity through which he could sneak into her mind and plant doubt. Had Satan started out by telling Eve that God was a liar, Eve probably would have had the good sense to laugh in his face and retort that *he's* the liar. But Satan is shrewd, and he knows our area of vulnerability, and that's exactly where he attacks first.

"Did God really say, 'You must not eat from any tree in the garden'?" he asks innocently (Genesis 3:1). What a ridiculous question! Adam and Eve had been enjoying the delicious fruits this whole time, and in their perfect relationship with God, they would have responded to this abundance with grateful hearts and words of praise. So Eve quickly corrects him.

"Of course we may eat fruit from the trees of the garden!" *Duh. What else do you think we've been doing this whole time?* she seems to imply. But rather than shake her head and walk away, Eve continues to engage the conversation, and that's exactly what this sneaky snake was looking for.

"It's only the fruit from the tree in the middle of the garden that we are not allowed to eat," she continues, and that seems to be a reasonable restriction. After all, she hadn't questioned it up to this point. "God said, 'You must not eat it or even touch it; if you do, you will die!'" Eve concludes.

At this point, it's good to step aside and compare Eve's summary of God's command with the actual command God gave Adam in Genesis 2:16–17 (NLT): "You may freely eat the fruit of every tree in the garden—except the tree of the knowledge of good and evil. If you eat its fruit, you are sure to die."

While Eve attempted to set the record straight, she belittled the privileges God had given her and her husband in several ways:

> She left out God's "freely eat," a phrase that speaks to God's generosity and the delight He took in His children's enjoyment of the food He had given them.

> She downplayed God's emphasis on their ability to eat fruit from every tree but one. In the grand scheme of things, the rule wasn't

depriving them of much considering the abundance of options they had to choose from.

She added the rule about not touching the fruit, which wasn't part of God's command.

Now we don't know if that extra rule about not touching the fruit came when Adam passed on the command to Eve or if Eve had made it for herself as a safeguard. You know, like when you reroute your way home from work so you won't drive past the donut shop and won't even be tempted to swing into the drive-through. We all add extra rules and restrictions for ourselves to keep us far away from trouble, and it's possible that's what happened here with Eve. But as we'll see, bad things happen when we downplay God's goodness and provision for us and elevate our own self-imposed rules to the level of God's commandments.

Back to the scene in the garden.

"You won't die!" the serpent reassured Eve. And she may have nodded in agreement, acknowledging that okay, really, touching the fruit wasn't the issue. But before she could reply and clarify God's command, Satan goes on, boldly negating God's clear command and consequences. "God knows that your eyes will be opened as soon as you eat it, and you will be like God, knowing both good and evil" (Genesis 3:5 NLT).

Hold on there.

What just happened?

Satan just called God a liar. And before Eve could even think of a response, Satan lured her with the promise of pleasures untasted and power unfettered.

Starting from that first apparently innocent question that Eve easily shot down, the serpent led Eve along a well-planned path, introducing doubt and causing her to ultimately question the goodness of God.

The result was devastating. Eve was convinced by the serpent's sly words and cunning logic. The next thing we know she's standing under the forbidden tree, looking at it longingly, noticing that "the tree was beautiful and its fruit looked delicious" (Genesis 3:6 NLT). Had she not seen the tree before? Of course she had. It was in the center of the garden. She had probably walked past that tree hundreds of times and hadn't given it a second thought. But now that she was entertaining doubt, she began wondering if God really was holding out on her. Maybe there was some truth to what the serpent had said.

Of course Satan is not more trustworthy than God. We should run as far away from him as we can.

Not only did she begin craving the forbidden fruit, she also began longing for "the wisdom it would give her" (v. 6 NLT). How did she know it would give her wisdom? Well, because the serpent said so. And he's certainly more credible than God Himself, the one who tenderly fashioned Adam and Eve and placed them in a garden of abundance with all they could ever want. Right? So she took some of the fruit, and ate it; and then she gave some to Adam, who apparently had been standing by passively the whole time.

Looking at Eve in that moment, it's easy to recognize where she went wrong. Of course Satan is not more trustworthy than

God. Of course we shouldn't take him at his word. Of course we should run as far away from him as we can. But what's so clear when we're removed from the situation becomes quickly muddled when we're caught up in our own little confrontations with lies.

Devastating Consequences

The enemy's lies aren't innocent. He's not out to amuse himself by pushing us around and having a good time. His goal is clear: Satan wants to destroy us.

The consequence of believing these lies isn't just a little slap on the wrist. For Adam and Eve, they received the penalty God assured them would happen—that day they experienced spiritual death, and physical death entered the world as well. All of creation suffered because of their choice to believe the enemy's lies.

And while our own encounters with lies may seem mild in comparison, the reality is that believing Satan's lies is just as devastating in our own lives today as it was in Eve's and Adam's lives that fateful day so long ago.

As we've already discovered, the enemy comes only to lie, kill, and destroy, and he will resort to whatever tactics he needs to accomplish his mission. In your own life, you may have already seen the consequences of believing his lies related to food.

> You may be experiencing severe health issues and life-threatening diseases because of your food choices.

You may have suffered strained relationships or heartbreaking situations due to your lack of self-control, exhibited in your eating and in other areas of your life.

You may question whether God is as powerful as He says He is, since He hasn't helped you change.

You may avoid inviting people over for dinner or being a guest in other people's homes because it's too difficult to accommodate dietary preferences.

You may feel hopeless about the future, convinced that you'll never amount to anything because you're held back by these crippling habits.

You may be so consumed by thoughts of eating healthy and avoiding the latest black-listed ingredients that you have little mental energy to think of anything else, and your food choices become the center of your universe.

But it doesn't have to be this way.

We don't need to cower in fear of the enemy's lies because we can fight his lies with truth.

Take Every Thought Captive

Travel with me to another garden. It's the night before Jesus' crucifixion, and He was giving His disciples His last instructions before His death. In a beautiful setting Jesus looks at His followers and says, "I am the way and the truth and the life" (John 14:6). No matter what would happen later that night, no matter how despondent their circumstances seemed, no matter what difficulties they would face in the future, those followers of Jesus could rest in the fact that Jesus was the real deal. And He was all they needed to not just get through life but to be victorious in their lives.

Seventy-eight times in the four Gospels, Jesus says, "I tell you the truth!" Whereas our enemy is the father of lies, Jesus speaks the truth because He *is* Truth Himself. Jesus cannot speak anything but truth because He is God, and God defines what is true and what is reality. The best Satan can do is try to distort and warp what God has spoken as true.

You may be familiar with the well-loved verse, "You will know the truth, and the truth will set you free" (John 8:32). This isn't just a philosophical proposition of truth. Jesus is speaking here about knowing truth by knowing God Himself. As we deepen our relationship with God, His words will reside in us, and His Truth will free us of the lies that held us captive to food fixation.

Let's go back to Paul's letter to the Corinthians and take a look at the next verse in this passage on spiritual warfare: "We demolish arguments and every pretension that sets itself up against the knowledge of God, and we take captive every thought to make it obedient to Christ" (2 Corinthians 10:5). According to Paul, the battle begins in our minds. Paul explains that we knock down any thought patterns that exalt themselves above the truth of God. Lies and half-truths have no place in the mind of a believer devoted to God.

As we begin examining thoughts, we quickly realize we need to know the Word of God in order to recognize lies from truth. His words are life-giving truths that we can cling to. They are promises that we can be assured will come true. And they are the representation of His very presence in our lives through Jesus Christ, the Word made flesh.

The only way to take down the stronghold of food fixation is to take captive every single thought and make it bow its knee to Jesus Christ. As we change our thoughts, filling our minds with God's Word, we will begin to see change in our behavior as well. As we think Christ's thoughts, we will live out His Word through the power of His Spirit alive in us.

Transformative Change

When it comes to defeating lies, it doesn't take much to begin seeing change. It's a simple three-step solution that, once learned, can become second nature. But it requires intentionality and thoughtfulness when you first start out. It is simply:

1. Dig Up the Lie

Instead of allowing our thoughts to run rampant and attack us from every side, we must take each thought captive. Just as a gardener carefully examines each green leaf in her plot and pulls out the weeds, so we learn to pay attention to each thought that crosses our minds and determine whether to keep or discard it. Ask yourself, "Does this thought align with what God says in Scripture? Is it true? Is it beneficial? Does it glorify God?" If the thought doesn't pass this simple test, then take it captive, document it (write it out in words so you can clearly verbalize the lie), and make it submissive to Christ.

2. Fill Up with Scriptural Truth

Once you've identified the lie, it's time to go to Scripture and seek the truth. What does God say about this thought? Where has this lie distorted truth? If you're not sure, using a concordance or a Bible index will help. You'll also find Twenty Scriptures to Overcome Food Fixation in the bonus section of this book.

This is a critical step, so don't overlook it. It's not enough to just identify the lie and then let it go wild. We must incapacitate the lie by replacing it with truth. Only by filling our minds and our homes with the words of God can we neutralize the scripts the enemy has been playing in our minds. Post meaningful verses around your home and read them out loud whenever you're tempted to believe a lie. Soon you will be quick to recognize the lie as soon as it enters your mind and you'll cut it down within seconds, without even thinking about it. It really is as easy as that. We exchange the lies we believe with the truth that sets us free, and as our thought life changes, so will our behaviors.

3. Grow Up in Mature Faith

As we fill our minds with God's Truth, His Word begins producing in us the fruit of righteousness. God explains that just as the rains water the seeds to produce a plentiful harvest, "so is my word that goes out from my mouth: it will not return to me empty, but will accomplish what I desire and achieve the purpose for which I sent it" (Isaiah 55:11). God's Word always accomplishes His purposes, and the Holy Spirit uses Scripture to transform our thoughts, behaviors, and experiences.

When we dig up lies and fill up with Scripture, we will grow up in mature faith, because over time new thought patterns lead to new behaviors. Mature faith is transformative faith—it's seeing the fruit of the Spirit (from love and joy all the way to self-control) becoming more evident in our lives. This is a life-long process of maturation, but we will see progress week by week and year over year until we reach full maturity in heaven.

Yes, the mental battle is tenacious and requires constant vigilance. But the war is already won. We need only to claim the victory that is ours in Christ Jesus, as we take every thought captive and make it submissive to Christ, replacing the enemy's lies with God's truth.

On the following pages you will find ten food lies we too often fall for, along with scriptural affirmations to help you grow up in mature faith.

Digest the Truth

(for individual or group response)

1. Do you ever avoid hard things in your life by running to food instead? As you take steps toward real comfort and satisfaction in Jesus, what will be the hardest changes to make? Why?

2. Which of the food lies we have discussed have you believed? Read Ten Lies about Food on the following pages. Can you add others? Describe what happens when you act in accordance with the lie.

3. What food lies are you most susceptible to? How can you catch yourself the next time so you don't fall for the same lie?

4. This week, what will you do to replace the enemy's lies with the Word of God?

Bonus Online Content

Download "The Full Life Thought Chart" at http://www.thefull.life/chart and "Fill Up Affirmations" at http://www.thefull.life/daily-affirmations.

Ten Lies about Food

What are the lies you most believe? As we engage this spiritual battle, we must first identify the food lies we believe and then renew our minds with God's Truth, which will change our behavior, creating new habits that honor God.

Here are ten common food lies many women believe and the root of those lies. Fill up instead on affirmations based on God's Word and practical ways you can act on those truths.

Lie 1: I deserve a treat!

Dig Up the Lie:

"I've had a hard day today. I can't believe everything I had to put up with! I need a treat. After all, I deserve it."

Fill Up with Scriptural Truth:

"This treat doesn't bring lasting happiness—only the Lord can satisfy me. What I really want, more than a treat, is the peace, freedom, and joy found only in Him."
(see Psalm 90:14)

"Breaking boundaries is not a reward. When I choose to celebrate with God and delight in Him, He gives me the peace and freedom my heart desires." (see Psalm 37:4)

"God is my reward, and I experience abundant life when I feast on Him instead of obsessing over my next bite. His presence is better than any treat." (see Matthew 4:4)

"When I achieve a milestone, I know that really God did it. I don't deserve anything but God showers me with blessings, so I will give God His due praise and worship Him." (see James 1:16–17)

Grow Up in Mature Faith:

Journal about why you feel like eating a treat and why you think you have a right to eat a treat. Describe what happens when you eat whatever you believe you deserve. What habits does that create?

Memorize and meditate on the passages referenced above.

Learn creative ways to celebrate your own success and show others love and affection that don't involve food. It can be personal such as a massage, manicure, or a new outfit; an outing; going out to a movie, show, or concert; hiking to a special place, taking in an amusement park, visiting a museum, exploring an antiques store or a flea market, or even taking a drive. Or write a card, give a hug. Do their chores for a day, take out the garbage, sweep the garage, do the laundry, make a special trip to the store. Make a handmade card or gift, or surprise them with a random act of kindness. The possibilities are endless!

Lie 2: I can eat whatever I want.

Dig Up the Lie:

"No one gets to tell me what I can and cannot eat. I'll eat whatever I feel like, thank you very much. An extra treat here or there doesn't matter."

Fill Up with Scriptural Truth:

"Just because I can doesn't mean I should. I will not be mastered by my lusts." (see 1 Corinthians 6:12)

"I choose to eat in a way that glorifies Jesus Christ, not for my own selfish desires." (see Colossians 3:17)

"What I eat impacts how I feel and how I live. I choose to eat what will make me strong, energetic, and fit for God's good work." (see Galatians 6:7–8)

"My stomach is not the boss of me. I'm destined for greater things." (see Philippians 3:19–20)

Grow Up in Mature Faith:

Memorize 1 Corinthians 6:12–13 and/or 1 Corinthians 6:19–20. Place these verses on your fridge, in your pantry, or anywhere else you'll see them when cravings hit.

Take care of the body God gave you by getting enough rest, choosing healthy foods, and exercising regularly. You wouldn't invite a guest to stay in a room full of junk, would you? You'd clean it up and make sure they feel comfortable. So treat your body as the prized living space of our amazing God.

Practice worshiping God with your body. Dedicate each body part to Him, starting from the top of your head to your toes, giving Him control of what you do with your hands, your mouth, your stomach, the places you go, and the things you do. Also try different worship postures, kneeling in prayer, lying prostrate before Him, lifting holy hands in praise, walking, running, or dancing. God created your body, and He said it was good. Give it back to Him in worship.

Lie 3: If a little is good, then a lot is better.

Dig Up the Lie:

"This tastes so good—I'm going to have one more bite. Mmm. Okay, one more, for good measure. Ah, whatever. There's only one piece left in the row. Might as well finish it off."

Fill Up with Scriptural Truth:

"Eating too much actually hurts me. I can enjoy this delicious food in moderation and celebrate God's goodness in every little bite." (see Proverbs 25:16)

"More isn't always better. I can enjoy God's gift of good food without becoming gluttonous." (see 1 Timothy 4:4, 8)

"Even though it seems hard to moderate how much I eat, being disciplined leads to the peaceful fruit of righteousness, and that's what I really want." (see Hebrews 12:11)

Grow Up in Mature Faith:

Fast from the food that tempts you to overeat. (For more on fasting, see chapter 5.)

When you feel tempted to overeat, remember the price that Jesus paid for you. Picture Him hanging on the cross, enduring agony, scorn, and shame to pay the price to redeem you from a life of despair. Refuse to despise such a great sacrifice of love by stuffing more food into your mouth, and instead turn your attention to worship.

Take the three-bite challenge. Researchers have discovered something called sensory specific satiety. Basically, our taste buds get numbed if they continually experience the same taste, so you experience less pleasure with each subsequent bite.[1] The next time you face your favorite treat, relish the first bite. Close your eyes and take the time to really enjoy the flavors. Turn your mind toward God and praise Him for inventing such a wide variety of foods, for giving you taste buds, and for providing the food before you. With your next bite, engage all five senses and let yourself fully experience the explosion of flavors. And with your third and last bite, direct your heart toward God once more, and ask Him to help you learn to enjoy Him as much as you enjoy that food.

Lie 4: I'll never overcome food fixation!

Dig Up the Lie:

"I've tried every program I can think of, and I'm not seeing any progress. This is just too hard! It's hopeless."

Fill Up with Scriptural Truth:

"God always provides a way out of tempting situations. I will run from food idolatry." (see 1 Corinthians 10:13–14)

"I can do all things through Christ who strengthens me." (see Philippians 4:13)

"I will not get discouraged in doing what is right, because in time I will reap the rewards if I don't give up." (see Galatians 6:9)

"I am confident that He who began a good work in me will complete it. He's not finished with me yet." (see Philippians 1:6)

"I haven't yet reached my goal, but I'm going to forget what's in the past and push forward to the victory that lies ahead in Jesus Christ." (see Philippians 3:13–14)

"Discipline is not easy but it's worth the struggle because after I've trained my body I will reap the peaceful fruit of righteousness." (see Hebrews 12:11)

"I can rejoice in this trial because it tests my faith and produces endurance, which will lead to being perfect and complete, lacking in nothing in Christ." (see James 1:2–4)

Grow Up in Mature Faith:

Memorize Galatians 6:9, Romans 8:11, Luke 1:37, and/or Philippians 4:13.

Continue living in obedience even when you don't feel like it. Create a healthy eating plan and stick with it. Don't base your eating choices on feelings; base them on what you *know* is true.

Get accountability. Find a friend who's on this journey with you and encourage each other when you're feeling down. Practice telling each other the lies that you've believed and send each other helpful Bible verses throughout the week.

Write down inspirational Bible verses or quotes. When you find a quote you like about self-discipline, God's view of food, or anything that you feel resonates with you during this journey, don't just skip over it: write it down! These words will come in handy when you're facing low motivation, and when you're tempted to forget why you're doing this in first place.

Lie 5: Just this once won't hurt.

Dig Up the Lie:

"Aw, come on. This is a special occasion. I'm going to indulge just this once, and I promise I'll do better tomorrow."

Fill Up with Scriptural Truth:

"It is for freedom that Christ has set me free. I'm going to stand firm and not get entangled in compromises."
(see Galatians 5:1)

"I will make no provision for the flesh. I'm not giving back a single inch of ground that I won in Jesus Christ."
(see Romans 13:14)

"I'm not going to get sloppy in this area of my life. I'm going to keep my eyes open and be smart about my food choices."
(see 1 Thessalonians 5:6)

Grow Up in Mature Faith:

Ban the phrase "I'll start tomorrow" from your vocabulary, acknowledging that you won't magically transform into a self-controlled person overnight. Discipline is fought for.

Write the phrase "today's decisions shape tomorrow's actions" somewhere you'll see it every day. We create habits one small bite at a time.

Decide ahead of time what treats and indulgences you'll allow yourself, and determine boundaries to protect you from overeating. For example, you might enjoy dessert only in the presence of others, or only on the weekend, or only if it's homemade. But whatever your personal boundaries are, stick with them.

Lie 6: Food will thrill me.

Dig Up the Lie:

"I'm so bored. There's nothing to do. I mean, yeah, there's that project I could work on, but I don't feel like doing it. I'll just grab a quick snack; *then* I'll get to work. This treat will hit the spot."

Fill Up with Scriptural Truth:

"God created food to nourish and energize me, not to entertain me. I'm going to find something better to do with my time." (see Genesis 9:3)

"I won't put off my work by grabbing a snack, because that snack won't help. But God will. With God, I can crush the assignments and jump over any obstacles." (see Psalm 18:29)

"If I avoid doing the work now, I'll still have to do it later. God, help me to be faithful in this task I have to do right now. Give me the strength and endurance to finish it well." (see Luke 16:10; Philippians 4:19)

Grow Up in Mature Faith:

Find something other than eating that you enjoy doing, and do that when you're bored. Make a list of fun activities that only take five or ten minutes, like painting your nails or going for a prayer walk until your craving passes.

Drink water. If you find you must snack on something while you work, keep a glass full of water at your side. Have fun infusing it with different fruits to keep it fresh.

When you want to eat out of procrastination, try breaking the project into smaller parts and working on your project for just ten minutes. Set a timer, and focus on your work. More often than not, you'll get into a groove and enjoy a productive session.

Lie 7: I can't let this food go to waste.

Dig Up the Lie:

"I feel kind of full, but there are only a few bites left. I can't let it go to waste—that's not good stewardship! I'll just clean up the plate so good food doesn't get thrown into the trash."

Fill Up with Scriptural Truth:

"I don't treat my body as a trashcan. It's the temple of the Holy Spirit. I will care for my body because it is the dwelling place of God." (see 1 Corinthians 6:19)

"Jesus purchased me—mind, body, and soul—with His own precious blood on the cross. I cherish Him by treating this body as His prized living space."
(see 1 Corinthians 6:20)

"God takes care of all my needs. I don't overeat because I trust Him to provide my next meal." (see Matthew 6:25–26)

Grow Up in Mature Faith:

Journal your responses to the following questions: Is eating extra food when you don't need it better than throwing it away? How does this type of behavior affect you in the long-term?

Think about some creative solutions: try serving smaller portions or saving leftovers to eat for lunch the next day.

Lie 8: I'll hurt her feelings if I don't eat what she offers.

Dig Up the Lie:

"She always serves a special treat when I come over. I don't really want to eat it, but I don't want to offend her either. What will she think of me? She'll be so hurt if I refuse."

Fill Up with Scriptural Truth:

"Perfect love casts out fear. This person loves me, and she wants what's best for me, including freedom from food fixation." (see 1 John 4:18)

"I live to please God, not others." (see Galatians 1:10; 1 Thessalonians 2:4; 2 Corinthians 5:9)

"Nothing can separate me from the love of God, even if someone else is disappointed in me." (see Romans 8:35–39)

Grow Up in Mature Faith:

When offered food that would break your boundaries, simply say, "No, thank you," and move on with the conversation. Don't make a big deal out of it, and chances are others won't either.

So many of our get-togethers center around food. If this frustrates you, then make the decision to host a gathering that doesn't involve food. It can be as simple as inviting some of your friends over for a painting party. Or hosting a prayer meeting and only serving tea. Other ideas include: going for a walk together, flea market or antique show, attending a lecture, going to an exercise or dance class, planting flowers, or volunteering.

Lie 9: Eating this will make me feel better.

Dig Up the Lie:

"I can't believe what happened today. I don't even want to think about it. Where's that secret stash I keep . . . there it is. This will make me feel better."

Fill Up with Scriptural Truth:

"Food cannot change my circumstances, but God can. Nothing is too difficult for Him." (see Genesis 18:14a)

"I only compound my misery when I take my brokenness to the fridge. Food cannot fix anything. God is the only one who can satisfy us because He created us to find our satisfaction in Him." (see Isaiah 58:11)

"I will not seek comfort in what doesn't satisfy. Instead, I will delight in the abundance found in God."
(see Isaiah 55:1–2)

"God promises me fullness of joy in His presence. I will turn away from comfort eating and feast in His presence instead." (see Psalm 16:11)

Grow Up in Mature Faith:

Buy a special notebook or journal to keep all your thoughts about your recovery in one place. Even though it's a little scary to put everything in writing, being 100 percent honest about your feelings is a challenge, but it's necessary. Acknowledge your feelings, relate what happened, and then write down the truth about who God says you are and the freedom He promises you as you push toward victory.

When's the last time you felt hungry? Describe the feeling. Did your stomach rumble? Did you get lightheaded? Whatever it is, write it down and put it on your fridge. The next time you look for something to eat, ask yourself if you're truly hungry.

Allow hunger—and not feelings—to determine when you eat. Think of physical fullness as a fuel gauge on your car: 3 is pleasantly full and 10 is overstuffed. Then think of physical hunger on the negative scale: -3 is kind of hungry and -10 is ravenous. Eat when you're at a -3 and stop when you're at a 3. Avoid the extremes.

Lie 10: I messed up, so I give up.

Dig Up the Lie:

"What a mess! I can't even stick to a healthy eating program. Oh, well. There's no point in even trying. I already blew it today, so I might as well go all-out. Pass the chips, please!"

Fill Up with Scriptural Truth:

"Father, I confess my sin to You. Thank You that You are faithful and just to forgive my sins and cleanse me from all unrighteousness." (see 1 John 1:9)

"Just because I messed up once doesn't mean I need to continue to sin. I died to sin, so I refuse to continue living in it." (see Romans 6:1–2)

"Jesus does not condemn me, so I will not condemn myself either. I will go and sin no more." (see John 8:10–11)

"I am not condemned by bondage to sin. The Spirit of Life has set me free from the law of sin and death."
(see Romans 8:1–2)

"I will trust God to save me from food fixation; it's God's gift from start to finish, so I won't brag about my victory. I will join Jesus Christ in this good work He's doing in my life."
(see Ephesians 2:8–10)

Grow Up in Mature Faith:

Celebrate small victories. If you stayed on plan for most of the day and blew it at dinner, thank God for helping you.

If you catch yourself in the middle of devouring a carton of ice cream, stop. Pour hot water over the remainder of the ice cream carton. Figure out how to get back on track, and move on.

Self-control is sometimes as easy as closing your mouth. Instead of thinking of your body as an all-you-can-eat buffet, think of it as a business that has office hours.

There's a sign on the front that says "open for business from 7–7:30 a.m., 12–12:30 p.m., and 5–5:30 p.m." All other times, the business, and your mouth, are closed. Don't allow food to enter your mouth during the hours your business is closed. It sounds simplistic, but it really works. Practice being mindful about what goes into your mouth. Business hours is just one way of doing that.

While you may not be able to stop these lies from entering your mind, you *can* keep from dwelling on them and acting on them. As Martin Luther said, "You can't stop the birds from flying over your head, but you can keep them from building a nest in your hair."

Consider this a starting point; over the next few days, identify the food lies you most often believe (whether they're on this list or not), and write out your own scripts based on Scripture. Soon you will change the way you think about food, and your actions will follow your thoughts.

Part Two

Awakening a
Desire for God

4

Stir Up a Holy Hunger

"*Read the Bible*, Mama!" she exclaimed as she ran toward me.

I looked up for a moment and then back down to my phone, finishing the eye-catching headline.

"READ!!" Her tone rose up a notch, and she shoved the children's illustrated Bible into my face, completely obstructing the glowing screen.

I looked up and met her gaze. Her eyes held a sort of urgency, and her jaw was set. At two years old, it would be easier to negotiate with a labor union leader than this little tyrant. And yet . . . I felt conviction prick my heart. It had been days since I had read my own Bible. A series of unfortunate events—ranging from pregnancy insomnia to my toddler's sleep regression to a collision of writing deadlines—combined to make me a tired, cranky, and not-fun-to-be-around mama, and honestly, the last thing I wanted was to sit down with my Bible only to be interrupted by my little one's clamoring.

But there she was, asking—no, *demanding*—that I read the Bible to her. She goes through phases, but David and Goliath was her favorite at the time. It didn't seem to matter that we had read that same story three times the day before; she didn't tire of hearing how this little boy gathered five smooth stones and went up against a big giant, defeating him in the name of his great God. She settled in my lap, careful not to disturb the baby bump, and laid her head against my shoulder.

"Read," she said again, quietly this time, anticipation lacing her words.

A Hunger for God

Throughout Scripture, men and women of God use the imagery of hunger and thirst to describe their desire for Him. David especially is well-known for his many psalms, my favorite of which is Psalm 63. As King David penned these words, he was in the desert, again fleeing for his life, most likely this time from his son Absalom.

All the comforts of the palace had been stripped away from him: delectable foods, wine, fluffy pillows, cool chambers, loving family. And in their place were blistering heat, whipping wind, stale bread, lukewarm water, and bloodthirsty pursuers. It is in this context that David calls out to God in verses 1–5:

> You, God, are my God,
>> earnestly I seek you;

I thirst for you,
>   my whole being longs for you,
in a dry and parched land
>   where there is no water.
I have seen you in the sanctuary
>   and beheld your power and your glory.
Because your love is better than life,
>   my lips will glorify you.
I will praise you as long as I live,
>   and in your name I will lift up my hands.
I will be fully satisfied as with the richest of foods;
>   with singing lips my mouth will praise you.

It is striking that in such dire conditions, bereft of all comforts and pleasures, David can still claim complete satisfaction in God; in God's presence he had found satisfaction "as with the richest of foods." Imagine the best fare a palace chef could cook. Picture your favorite meal. Look up the menus at the world's most prestigious restaurants. They don't even compare to the satisfaction found in God's presence, David says. Those who hunger and thirst for God will be satisfied.

And it's not just Psalm 63 where David makes these claims. Look at how Scripture speaks of being satisfied in God:

>   You make known to me the path of life; in
>   your presence there is fullness of joy; at your
>   right hand are pleasures forevermore.
>   —Psalm 16:11 ESV

>   I have learned to be content whatever the
>   circumstances. I know what it is to be in

need, and I know what it is to have plenty. I
have learned the secret of being content in
any and every situation, whether well fed or
hungry, whether living in plenty or in want.
I can do all this through him who gives me
strength. —Philippians 4:11–13

I call on you, my God, for you will answer
me; turn your ear to me and hear my prayer.
... I will be vindicated and will see your face;
when I awake, *I will be satisfied with seeing
your likeness*. —Psalm 17:6, 15

You open your hand and satisfy the desires of
every living thing. —Psalm 145:16

God [created humans] so that *they would seek
him and perhaps reach out for him and find him*,
though he is not far from any one of us. "For
in him we live and move and have our being."
—Acts 17:27–28a

Blessed are those who hunger and thirst for
righteousness, for they shall be satisfied.
—Matthew 5:6 ESV

This last verse is worth pausing on for a moment, because it clearly states a prerequisite to finding satisfaction in
God, namely this: In order to be satisfied in God, we must first
hunger and thirst for Him.

The Greek word for *blessed* here means "the highest good,
to be supremely blessed, happy, fortunate, well off."[1] It's interesting here that Jesus ties together satisfaction to our hunger

and thirst for righteousness. He's saying that if we're craving anything else, we will never really experience true satisfaction. No matter how much we eat, no matter how many cookies, how many buffet lines, how many late-night escapades, we will never truly be satisfied as long as we are craving something other than Him.

If we desire God, if we hunger and thirst for righteousness, He promises that not only will we get to taste His goodness, but that we will be satisfied. The Greek word for *satisfied* here actually means "to gorge."[2] This is surprising to me, because gorging has always carried with it a negative connotation. We have probably all experienced at least one time in our lives when we gorged on food, when we tasted something that was so good that we kept eating and lost all control, until we had more than we could take. Jesus is using this exact word to help us picture the immense satisfaction that is ours in God when we hunger and thirst for Him instead of empty food. That's mind-blowing to think about.

I read Matthew 5:6 early in my journey toward overcoming food fixation. Right there, in the middle of the day, right where I was sitting in the sunroom with my Bible open, I began praying earnestly, "Lord, if I'm completely honest, I don't really hunger for You. I don't thirst for You. I'm okay doing my own thing, but I don't want to live this way anymore. Give me a

God created us to know Him, to enjoy Him, and to be loved by Him. And when we spend time in His presence, He changes us, creating in us a desire to grow even closer to Him.

hunger and thirst for You. Change my cravings from food to You. Amen."

I opened my eyes, expecting something dramatic to happen . . . but nothing did. No light streamed from heaven, no fire burned in my heart, and no change took place inside me. I shut the Bible, disheartened and ready to give up. But the next morning, I showed up for my quiet time in the sunroom again, and I prayed that same prayer and added, "Deeper, Lord. I want to go deeper with You. Do whatever it takes to shake me from this apathy, and awaken a hunger within me."

Day after day, I'd show up and pray that simple prayer, clinging to God's promise to make Himself known to those who seek Him. And little by little, He began kindling in me a hunger for Him. God created us to know Him, to enjoy Him, and to be loved by Him. And when we spend time in His presence, He changes us, creating in us a desire to grow even closer to Him.

Throughout the Bible, God invites us to bring our requests to Him, even expecting us to approach Him in His throne room with boldness, because Jesus speaks on our behalf (Hebrews 4:16). So we are confident that we will receive whatever we ask for according to His will, because God says so (1 John 5:14).

But God's promise doesn't mean that He will answer our selfish prayers for a smaller waist or a faster metabolism. Believe me, I've tried it. Maybe you have too. He doesn't work that way. When we pray from selfish desires to match our society's standards of beauty or to give our appetites free rein, we're simply rubbing the proverbial genie bottle with no effect. A selfish prayer with the words "in Jesus' name" won't magically be answered. God is not in the business of fulfilling selfish wishes.

After all, "prayer keeps us in constant communion with God, which is the goal of our entire believing lives. Without a doubt, prayerless lives are powerless lives, and prayerful lives are powerful lives; but believe it or not, the ultimate goal God has for us is not power but personal intimacy with Him."[3] Instead, when we center our prayers on pleasing Him with our lives, we are guaranteed to receive what we ask for in prayer, because He answers prayers that are rooted in His character.

I can't point to any specific instance and say "*That's* when I began hungering for God." I just know that as I sought Him with all my heart, He rewarded me with more of Himself. The more I hungered, the more He satisfied; and the more He satisfied, the more insatiable my appetite became.

When We Don't Desire God

God delights in awakening our spiritual hunger if we ask Him to do so and submit our lives to Him. Praying for a deeper relationship with God, a greater hunger for His presence, a release from anything that distracts us from Him pleases God, because it's what He wants for us too. And when we pray for these things, He quickens to answer, satisfying us with Himself "as with the richest of foods" (Psalm 63:5).

Look again at the Sermon on the Mount in Matthew 5; Jesus says that those who hunger and thirst for God are blessed because they get to eat and drink their fill of Him and never go unsatisfied again. This blessing isn't reserved for the elite few—it's available to anyone who cries out to Him in desperation, longing to be satisfied with His presence.

But what if we don't? What if, when we're honest with ourselves, we admit that we crave chocolate chip cookie dough more than communion with the Creator? What if we'd rather bake up a treat than bask in His presence? What if we recognized that we'd rather stuff down our feelings with Oreos than face our pain with our Savior?

I think we're often afraid of admitting our indifference toward God, for fear that He will strike us dead. But think of it—God already knows the state of our hunger (or lack thereof) for Him. We won't impress or disappoint Him by being truthful, but we will begin making headway when we are honest.

So this is where we must start: we must examine our spiritual appetites for God and honestly assess ourselves. And as we do so, we must ask the Spirit to shine His light in our hearts, because we can so easily deceive ourselves, thinking we're better off than we really are. But like David, we must pray, "Search me, God, and know my heart; test me and know my anxious thoughts. See if there is any offensive way in me, and lead me in the way everlasting" (Psalm 139:23–24).

Too many Christians don't hunger for God because they're too preoccupied with food. But it's only when we're sincere about our spiritually dormant appetites that we can be awakened to His glorious sufficiency. Here are a few questions, inspired by several passages of Scripture, to help us gauge our hunger for God:

> When faced with a difficult situation, am I
> more likely to pause and pray, or postpone a
> decision by grabbing a bite to eat?
> —Acts 17:27–28a

After a long day, do I reward myself with a
treat, or with time in God's presence?
—Psalm 17:15

When circumstances are difficult in my life,
do I seek comfort in food, or in God's Word?
—Psalm 119:143

Do I more often feel the rumble of physical or
spiritual hunger? —Matthew 5:6

When I first wake up in the morning, do I
rush to check my phone, or do I open my
Bible? —Lamentations 3:22–24

Am I more likely to crave a snack, or a few
moments of silence with God?—Psalm 145:16

When someone takes the last serving of my
favorite dessert, do I get annoyed, or do I
smile contentedly? —Philippians 4:11–13

What brings me greater joy: a surprise gift
card to my favorite restaurant, or a surprise
extra hour to spend in worship? —Psalm 16:11

The point here is not that food, eating, or dining at restaurants is bad. On the contrary, these are good gifts from our
loving Father. But even good gifts can woo the heart away from
the Giver, and become idols in themselves. And when they
are, they must be swiftly removed or else risk them suffocating
any desire for God at all. Amy Carmichael knew this well. As a
single missionary to India at the turn of the last century, Amy
was disheartened to realize that many missionaries had left the
comfort of their homes only to seek the same comforts in their

lives abroad, often at the cost of their Christian witness. She realized the dangers of these simple things, and challenged her colleagues with these words:

> Comrades in this solemn fight . . . Let us settle it as something that cannot be shaken: we are here to live holy, loving, lowly lives. We cannot do this unless we walk very, very close to our Lord Jesus. Anything that would hinder us from the closest walk possible to us till we see Him face to face is not for us.[4]

Like Amy, we too must step away from anything that threatens a close walk with God. If you've answered those questions above and found your hunger for God lacking, do not be discouraged. That is good news, friend! For recognizing our apathy toward God is the very first step in this journey.

A hunger for God cannot be fabricated or imitated—it's the result of a personal encounter with the living Bread of Life. But I've discovered there are things we can do to make ourselves available to Him. In my own life, God used prayer, fasting, His Word, and worship to awaken my hunger for Him, and it's been an incredible journey so far. So if we do not, at the moment, hunger for God, we must ask Him to stir up our appetites for Him.

Stuffed with Good Gifts

Growing up a pastor's kid and later a missionary kid, I was familiar with the parable of the sower and the seed. It's a great story, often used in evangelistic contexts, and basically goes like this: A farmhand goes out to scatter seed onto the land. Some of the seed falls on the hardened ground of a pathway; some falls on rocky ground; some falls among the tall weeds; and yet some other seed falls on fertile soil. (For the full parable, see Luke 8:4–15.)

The point of the story is that you want to be that last type of ground: the fertile soil, where God's Word can grow and produce a crop.

And for the better part of my life, I was convinced that's the soil I was. After all, I had grown up in church, I had accepted Jesus as my Savior when I was a child, I had surrendered my life to God when I was a teenager, and I had served Him throughout my life alongside my family. There was no doubt I was good soil.

But the summer God began working in my life on this issue of food fixation, I read this parable with new eyes. My gaze lingered on Luke 8:14, and it struck me as if I had never read it before: "The seed that fell among thorns stands for those who hear, but as they go on their way they are choked by life's worries, riches and pleasures, and they do not mature."

Certainly, there had been seasons in my life when my heart was good soil, when the Word produced a crop in my life not just in my deeds but in my devotion. But to be honest, I had been stagnating in my faith as of late, and there was little to no desire for God. Sure, I still did all the right things. I prayed, read the Bible, went to church, and served in young adult ministries. I had even started a Christian blog not too long before.

But that day I realized that I had allowed "life's worries, riches and pleasures" to grow wild in my heart, and they had choked the Word of Life. As I sat with my journal, I listed the things that had been preoccupying me over the previous months, and the list read ugly but honest: obsessed with losing the baby weight; worried about our finances; anxious about eating the right foods; envious about other people's success; preoccupied with my blog's growth; nervous about my husband's job.

At the same time, I had allowed life's simple pleasures to woo me away from wholehearted devotion to God: I was baking treats two or three times a week instead of spending that time in God's Word; I was eating sweets instead of healthy meals; I was binge-watching TV shows instead of worshiping God; I was reading pointless articles instead of inspiring biographies about godly people; I was staying up late at night endlessly scrolling through my Facebook feed instead of going to bed early to meet with the Lord in the morning. My life was a disorganized mess, and I had allowed my desires to dictate my actions. The thorny weeds had grown from innocent little tufts here and there to monstrosities overrunning the garden, and there was no way I could uproot them on my own.

I stopped praying for a smaller waist and faster metabolism and began praying, "Deeper, Lord. Take me deeper into Your presence."

The pleasures that drove me were reckless taskmasters, and I discovered that my desires were entirely misplaced. Faced with the terrible truth of my weedy heart-garden, I fell on my knees before God. *Dear Lord*, I whispered. *This is worse than I imagined. I didn't even realize all these sins were in my heart, let alone growing all over the place. I'm so sorry. And I feel so overwhelmed. Where do I even start?! Forgive me, Father. Till up the soil of my heart. Dig down deep and pull out the thorny weeds by the root; leave nothing of the old. Till up my heart, Lord, and let it be fertile ground for You.*

Immediately, the Spirit of God revealed to me drastic changes I had to make in my life, if I truly desired to see change. I stopped watching those shows which, though not inherently bad, were sucking up my time. I made a daily appointment with the Lord for prayer, worship, and Bible study, and I kept it. I deleted the Facebook, Twitter, and Pinterest apps from my phone. I placed Christian classics in my living room, so they would be within easy reach when I had a few moments of free time. I scribbled verses on sticky notes and placed them around the house—inside cabinet doors, on the fridge, over the sink, and in the bathroom. I unsubscribed from marketing newsletters and podcasts that caused me anxiety and worry because I wasn't doing enough with my blog, and I invited silence into my life instead. I listened for the Spirit's voice when I ran to the shelf for cookies and put them back, hitting my knees in prayer to talk about whatever drove me to food in the first place. I stopped praying for a smaller waist and faster metabolism and began praying, *Deeper, Lord. Take me deeper into Your presence.*

That season, though it lasted only a few weeks, was intense, and it stoked within me a hunger for God like I had never felt before. And ironically, I discovered that the more I feasted on God, the hungrier for Him I became. He began to fill me with His presence, and yet I wanted more. I realized the truth of John Piper's words, jotted in my notebook during this season:

> If you don't feel strong desires for the manifestation
> of God, it is not because you have drunk deeply and

are satisfied. It is because you have nibbled so long at the table of the world. Your soul is stuffed with small things, and there is no room for the great. God did not create you for this. There is an appetite for God. And it can be awakened.[5]

I Surrender All

As we confess those small things that have stuffed our souls, God will be faithful to uproot them and make room for His great presence. But beware, God is not content with merely the trifles we offer Him—He wants *all* of us. Like my sweet friend Wendy shared of her forty-day sugar fast: "God said to me, 'thanks for the sugar, but *I want all of you.*'"

You may have heard the saying "Jesus is either Lord of all or He's not Lord at all," and there's truth to that. We cannot pick and choose what we give God control over. There comes a point in each of our lives when we must make the decision: either we submit everything we are to all He is or we continue living lives of quiet desperation, seeking satisfaction in all the empty promises of half-full peanut butter jars and candy bags.

Speaking of His followers Jesus said, "I have come that they may have life, and have it to the full" (John 10:10). Did you catch that? *Life to the full.* Jesus didn't leave His disciples to wonder what type of life they would have with Him—He wanted them to be certain. Life with Jesus is full: full of joy in His presence, full of the riches of His glory, full of comfort in sufferings, full of rejoicing in hardships, full of pleasures at His right hand, full of life in this world and the next.

We get *the full life*, not just the physical sensation of feeling full after a good meal, which is what most people want (and most dieters don't get) but something that is deeper and more satisfying than the most delicious feast. Jesus wants us to experience the fullness that comes only from Him. A satisfaction that permeates all of life; that is what we actually long for when we turn to food but will never find outside of Jesus. But this fullness will only come once we have renounced anything that would compete with Him in our affections.

We must examine what threatens our wholehearted devotion to God, and lay it down on the altar, entrusting it to Him. Having given God our sweet tooth, our food fixation, our obsession with looking thin or fit or stylish, our desire to control our health by eating healthy—whatever that idol was that caused us to obsess—having laid that on the altar, we must ask, *What else, God? What else threatens to squelch my desire for You? Take it all.*

Though this uprooting of sins hurts, it's a healing operation, like removing a cancerous tumor that threatens one's life. We invite the pain of denying our own comforts and pleasures, our cravings and our whims, to experience a deeper hunger and thirst for Him. We surrender all we have to receive in exchange all He is, even His own kingdom. For Jesus also said, "Blessed are the poor in spirit, for theirs is the kingdom of heaven" (Matthew 5:3). But "till we are poor in spirit, Christ is never precious. Before we see our own wants, we never see Christ's worth."[6] So with quiet confidence we ask God to *take it all.*

> *We need only to ask, and He will awaken in us a spiritual hunger like we've never experienced before.*

If you're in that place right now, conscious of how insufficient your food idols have been and desperate for the presence of God in your life, put down this book and tell Him. Use your own words or the prayer I prayed, but whatever you do—don't continue life as usual until you have this face-to-face conversation with God. Tell Him you want more of Him. You're desperate for Him. You're not willing to live the rest of your life in a superficial relationship with Him. Tell Him you want the fullness of His presence in your life, just as He created you to experience in the first place.

And if you don't yet hunger for God? Tell Him that too. Be honest with Him, and tell Him you don't hunger for Him, but you *want* to want Him. He gets it. And your honesty won't scare Him away; if anything, it will help you recognize that you need His intervention to even *want to want Him.* Ask Him to make you famished for His presence. And keep praying until He answers. We need only to ask, and He will awaken in us a spiritual hunger like we've never experienced before.

If you don't see changes right away, take heart. God's working on His own timetable. Keep praying, and keep a humble heart before Him. God rewards all who diligently seek Him (Hebrews 11:6). And much like a toddler clamoring for *one more Bible story*, we too can experience the insatiable appetite of hungering for God. And, like David, we can experience God's presence as more desirable than even the finest chocolate.

Digest the Truth
(*for individual or group response*)

1. Read Psalm 63. In what ways does this psalm describe your desire for God's presence? In what ways is it different from what you currently desire?

2. How has your view of food influenced your view of God? How has your view of God influenced your view of food?

3. Does calling food fixation a sin make you uncomfortable? Have you confessed this sin to God? What are the benefits of confession? What are the dangers of not confessing?

4. Imagine yourself living the full life that Jesus talks about in John 10:10. What would that look like? How would you relate to food? How would you relate to God? What's keeping you from living that full life?

5. Do you believe God can really satisfy you more than food can? If no, why not? If yes, what are the implications of choosing God over food? What are the implications of choosing food over God?

Bonus Online Content
Watch Asheritah share about "When You Desire God Less Than You Thought," and download a worksheet to assess your hunger for God at http://www.thefull.life/heart-check.

Monica's story

By the time I was thirty-two, I had spent half of my life consumed with three things: food, exercise, and my body. Having been a gymnast growing up, I had been trained to count calories, track body fat, and exercise religiously. As I entered my teen and young adult years, I wanted so much to be free from this obsession. I searched for help—diets, exercise plans, or anything that might guide me through this daily wrestling match to find a way to live at peace with myself.

Finally, after my second son was born, I was determined to find another way to live. I laid down my burdens before the Lord and prayed for His help getting to the root of the problem. He showed me that I had believed lies about myself and my body. With His help, I began to focus my efforts on changing the way I thought. I got radical about banishing thoughts that were obsessive or negative, and replacing them with Scripture, positive affirmation, and truth. I trusted my body to let me know when I needed food, how to exercise moderately, and how to think differently.

It felt like a miracle when things began to change. As I embraced new thoughts, my behaviors changed, and it was not long before I found myself at my ideal weight. I have continued to practice this same way of thinking for nearly fourteen years. I had two more kids, and my weight has always returned to the same place. I have great faith that Christ's freedom is available to everyone in this area of struggle.[1]

5

Experience the Power of Fasting

As I prayed for God to awaken my hunger for Him, He brought me to Psalm 73:25–26: "Whom have I in heaven but you? And earth has nothing I desire besides you. My flesh and my heart may fail, but God is the strength of my heart and my portion forever."

I asked myself if that was true of my life. What had my utmost allegiance? What did I desire more than anything else on earth?

My simple answer, without batting an eyelash, had always been "God." I had read this psalm and even underlined it in several Bibles throughout the years, affirming with the psalmist that "God is my portion." He is enough.

But as God revealed my spiritual apathy, I wondered if that was really true or just wishful thinking. Could I test the limits of my satisfaction in Him? Was there a way to increase my desire for Him?

God showed me there is, and He led me to the discipline of fasting.

Fasting—What It Is (and Isn't)

Let's get something straight from the get-go: fasting is not a magic bullet. It's not a secret technique that will ensure permanent weight loss and an enviable figure. It's not even a surefire way to stir up a permanent hunger for God.

Nope.

Scripture teaches that the pursuit of holiness is a joint venture between God and believers. We are utterly dependent on God to work, yet God will not force a transformation on us without our inviting Him to do so. Fasting is one way to extend that invitation.

> *Fasting is an object lesson taught by the Spirit of God, helping us learn that we were created to find satisfaction in God alone.*

Fasting, when done scripturally, invites God to upend our lives, casting out idols we have allowed to woo us with their promises of comfort and satisfaction and reinstating the only source of satisfaction, which is God Himself.

Fasting isn't just not eating. That's called a diet, and a very bad one at that. Fasting is an object lesson taught by the Spirit of God, helping us learn that we were created to find satisfaction in God alone. In its simplest form, fasting is abstaining from food (or any other controlling substance or habit) for a set period of time for spiritual purposes. This discipline, when paired with prayer, can reveal the measure of food's mastery over us (or TV, the Internet, blogs, money, relationships, etc.).

In other words, fasting is intimacy expressed through forfeiting a good gift out of hunger for God; it puts our appetites to test and, if necessary, to death.

Fasting was practiced in both pagan and Jewish cultures, and was continued by the church throughout the past millennia. Some of the fasts we see appearing in the Bible, and that we can choose to practice in our own lives, are as follows:

> **Normal fast:** abstaining from all food but not from water (see Jesus' forty-day fast in the desert, Luke 4:2)
>
> **Partial fast:** abstaining from certain foods (see Daniel's diet restriction, Daniel 10:3)
>
> **Absolute fast:** abstaining from both food and water (see Esther and the Persian Jews' fast, Esther 4:16)
>
> **Supernatural absolute fast:** abstaining from both food and water for more than three days (see Moses's and Elijah's supernatural fasts, Exodus 24:18; 1 Kings 19:8)[1]

In other words, there's no one way to fast; it's a highly individualized experience between you and God (or, occasionally, a group of people and God—see Esther's corporate fast in Esther 4:16 and other public fasts in Leviticus 23:27). There are many reasons to fast, and Scripture shows us plenty of godly men and women who fast for everything from seeking God's guidance to expressing repentance, but in all those purposes, the one constant is inviting God to root out foreign affections and till up the soil of our hearts so that God's Word may produce its deserved fruit.[2] As such, fasting continues to be an essential discipline in the Christian's life and one Jesus assumed would be regularly practiced by the disciples in His absence.

Precautions in Fasting

While fasting is biblical and it is a method through which God often chooses to draw us closer into His presence, we must be careful to avoid some of the common pitfalls. Remember that the goal of fasting is not willpower or weight loss but worship, so whenever we engage in a fast, we must ask the Spirit to search our hearts and convict us of wrong reasoning. Truly, He is the one who teaches us how to practice this discipline in a way that leads to life and not to death.

> In the heart of the saint, both eating and fasting are worship. Both magnify Christ. Both send the heart—grateful and yearning—to the Giver. Each has its appointed place, and each has its danger. The danger of eating is that we fall in love with the gift; the danger of fasting is that we belittle the gift and glory in our willpower.[3]

Beware of fasting without repentance and humility.

Throughout the Old Testament, the Israelites practiced regular fasts, sometimes as often as twice a week. But speaking through His prophets, God informs them that their fasts are pointless: "Although they fast, I will not listen to their cry; though they offer burnt offering and grain offerings, I will not accept them. Instead, I will destroy them with the sword, famine and plague" (Jeremiah 14:12; see also Zechariah 7:5 and Isaiah 58:3).

Though the people went through external rituals, in their hearts they followed after false gods, worshiping idols, and embracing abominable practices, including child sacrifice, oppression of the poor, and extortion of the land. While we may not have those specific sins in our lives, the point here is that the attitude of our hearts and the testimony of our lives is more important than the ritual of fasting or any other discipline. We must live in genuine repentance and humility, or our fast is void.

If we approach fasting to break the bonds of food fixation, we must invite God to examine our hearts as we embark on a fast. Take some time in quiet prayer to ask God: What sins in my life do I need to repent of? In what ways have I treasured this thing I'm fasting of more than I've treasured You? What prideful tendencies do I need to be aware of as I start this fast?

If you can, write down these questions in a journal and wait expectantly. Write down the words, images, and situations that God brings to mind. Check them against Scripture. Talk to a trusted friend about them. Allow this fast to be the entry point for God to do His work in your life.

Beware of fasting to impress others.

You've seen those posts. You may have even posted one yourself: "I won't be on Facebook for the next few weeks because I'm fasting from social media for Lent." Is that kind of proclamation self-defeating?

When teaching His disciples about fasting, Jesus told them,

When you fast, do not look somber as the hypocrites do, for they disfigure their faces to show others they are fasting. Truly I tell you, they have received their reward in full. But when you fast, put oil on your head and wash your face, so that it will not be obvious to others that you are fasting, but only to your Father, who is unseen; and your Father, who sees what is done in secret, will reward you. (Matthew 6:16–18)

The Pharisees of Jesus' day had a small problem: they enjoyed showing off their spiritual prowess. Perhaps they wanted to inspire others to follow their example. Or maybe they were just following their mentors' example of fasting. But regardless, they wanted to impress others with their spirituality. And if I'm being honest, I've been guilty of this myself. Whether it's a shot of an open Bible, notebook, and morning mocha, or a trumpeted declaration of a Facebook fast, we've all maneuvered to make ourselves look just a little better in others' eyes.

According to Jesus, that's all the reward we will get. And really? Are a few Facebook likes and kudos what we're after? We should be seeking deep heart change, and that's not going to come from sharing our efforts for the whole world to see.

Does this mean that we never talk about our fast with others? Not necessarily. Sometimes it's helpful to speak of our fast to explain our actions, and when done with a contrite and humble heart, our sharing points to the surpassing goodness of God and gives Him glory. The point here is not to avoid talking about our fast altogether but rather to check our motives and make sure we're not just trying to impress.

As you think about and plan your fast, consider inviting others to participate with you. For two years in a row, I've joined a forty-day sugar fast, and the support, prayers, and accountability in that group were invaluable as we pushed one another to find satisfaction in Christ. Corporate fasts can be a great way to rally together in a discipline that is often neglected and misunderstood. Just make sure you're not doing it for the wrong reasons.

Beware of fasting as destructive bondage.

While some Christians have ignored fasting altogether, others would transform this discipline into a kind of asceticism that exalts fasting over feasting. Of these people, Paul warns in 1 Timothy 4:1–5 that "some will abandon the faith and . . . abstain from certain foods." The point Paul is making here is not that fasting is unbiblical but rather that a simplistic view of fasting can enslave people in a "harsh treatment of the body" that does not please God (see Colossians 2:23) but only results in exchanging carnal desires for diabolical self-reliance.

If we're not careful, fasting can become a form of bondage. Some of us who come from legalistic backgrounds were told that we *must* fast at a certain frequency, in specific ways in order to secure God's good favor. Nothing could be further from the truth. God will love us no more and no less whether we fast or not. His good graces have been secured by Jesus Christ on the cross, and nothing we can do could add or take away from that. Beware of anyone who teaches that fasting will make God more pleased with you. If you are a believer in Jesus, you are

Whenever we find our thoughts fixated on the foods we've given up during a fast, we must beg God to help us be consumed with thoughts of Him.

already preapproved; everything we do flows out of a place of spiritual rest, not restlessness.

Another destructive extreme in fasting is becoming so preoccupied with the food we're *not* eating that those foods consume our thoughts, taking our attention off of God and fixating it firmly on the food we're giving up. This is food fixation at its finest, masquerading as a spiritual discipline but actually working to undermine our hunger for God. As you fast, remember that giving up food is merely an external demonstration of what we desire to happen in our hearts. Whenever we find our thoughts fixated on the foods we've given up during a fast, we must beg God to help us be consumed with thoughts of Him.

While we're on this topic, a word about those who don't eat because of an eating disorder like anorexia nervosa. While this may technically be considered fasting, it's clearly not what God intended for us when He provided the biblical precedents of fasting. God gave us food as a good gift, and one way of worshiping God is receiving food with thanksgiving. As we've discussed, food is not the enemy. If you're struggling with an eating disorder, please seek help. God wants you to be free from this way of thinking.

Beware of fasting against medical advice.

This last cautionary point is more commonsense than explicitly biblically based, but it's important nonetheless.

When fasting, we must carefully consider our season of life and our medical history. For example, if you have a medical condition that requires you to eat at regular intervals to regulate your blood sugar, you would be wise to heed your doctor's advice and do so. Consider other kinds of fasts, like abstaining from certain junk foods or hobbies that dominate your time and affection. I've never heard of a medical condition that requires one to eat Cheetos and ice cream every day. If you can't do a normal fast (as defined above), consider a partial fast under your doctor's supervision.

Likewise, if you're pregnant or nursing, you are responsible to care for the child that is dependent on you for sustenance; abstaining from all food may harm not only your health but your baby's as well. This is a beautiful season of life and will be over shortly; during this time, ask God in what other ways you can fast to experience spiritual renewal.

And lastly, if you're considering an absolute fast (no food or water), prayerfully seek God's direction first. God created our bodies with very clear limitations, and our need for food and water to survive is one of them. Absolute fasts are the exception in Scripture, not the rule, and shouldn't be engaged in unless you have a very clear command from God, and then for no more than three days. A few years ago, a very dear elderly woman with multiple medical conditions undertook an absolute fast against her doctor's orders. She didn't eat or drink anything for seven days, and on the seventh day she had a stroke that left her incapacitated for the rest of her life. God has us here on earth for a reason, and we need to take good care of our bodies to serve Him here. For this reason, please consult your doctor before undertaking an extreme fast.

Turning Fasting into Feasting

Not all fasting is abstinence, however. An aspect of this practice that is often overlooked, but is crucial to our spiritual growth, is this: fasting is an opportunity to turn from the empty pleasures of this world and feast on the eternal pleasures of God Himself. As Corrie ten Boom put it: "You can never learn that Christ is all you need until Christ is all you have."[4]

All those who believe in Jesus are invited to feast on Him and, in so doing, to discover the source of true fullness. None of the momentary pleasures we experience can compare to the surpassing greatness of knowing Jesus personally, intimately, and sufficiently. And by this I mean a personal experience in which you realize that Jesus, the One you love and adore, is sufficient.

I invite you to participate in some simple fasts and keep your heart and mind focused not on what you're giving up but on what you're gaining. Take captive those thoughts of donuts and salted caramel truffles; let them drive you to your knees and declare, "This much, O Lord, I want You! As my body craves sugar and my mind is consumed with thoughts of food, I want my heart to be consumed by a hunger for You!"

Learning to Fast for God

As we remember that fasting is first and foremost a means of worship, we can approach this spiritual discipline as a learned discipline. Just as a child learns single-syllable words before forming sentences and coherent logical arguments, so we also learn the rudiments of fasting before we engage in some of the fasting feats we read about in books.

Here are some practical tips for fasting:

Determine beforehand what your fast will look like.

There are many ways to fast, and you may find yourself gravitating toward different fasts in different seasons of life. Prayerfully ask yourself what your goal is in fasting, and determine what kind of fast will help you in that. You may decide to fast from food once a week for the foreseeable future; in doing so, you'll be joining thousands of Christians around the world who practice this spiritual discipline on a regular basis. Or perhaps you'll decide to engage in a short-term fast, either by yourself or with your local church, like an Advent or Lenten fast. Whatever you decide, be clear what your fast will be like and how you will pursue fullness in God.

Begin with a slow progression.

If you're new to fasting, considering starting with a twenty-four-hour partial fast from lunch one day to lunch the next, once a week for several weeks. This means you're abstaining from dinner and breakfast, which is doable for a healthy adult. You may want to drink fresh fruit and vegetable juices during the fast, as you train your body to go without solid foods.

Fix your heart on Christ.

During your fast, you'll be tempted to bemoan all the foods you can't eat or the activities you can't partake in because of your fast. Resist the temptation to make this fast about what you must do without and instead focus on what you have the privilege of feasting upon. Remember that the point of the fast isn't just to make it to the end without eating; the point is to turn our hearts toward God in worship and learn to feast on Him instead. Cultivate a spirit of worship, prayer, and adoration, doing every task with a renewed sense of purpose as an act of service to the Lord.

Break your fast with worship and introspection.

Before you break your fast, journal your experience and any insights you have gained. Reflect on which Scriptures the Spirit brought to mind and how they informed your conduct. Confess and repent of the sins revealed during the fast. Think about the ways you were tempted and how God sustained you. Spend a few minutes worshiping God, praising Him for being the Bread of Life and any other attribute that comes to mind. As week follows week, you'll notice a progression in your journaling as well, as you go deeper in your reflections of who God is and what He's doing in your life.

Ease into eating.

If you engaged in a normal fast, end your fast with a light meal of fresh fruits and vegetables, rejoicing in God's gift of good food and His provision in other areas of your life as well. Resist the temptation to overeat everything you couldn't have the previous hours. Instead, use this meal as a reminder that we do not "live on bread alone" and that our real food that sustains us is to do God's work (John 4:32, 34).

Allow your first experiences with fasting to humble you. You don't need to get it perfect from the start. You might pop a handful of M&Ms in your mouth before you remember that you were supposed to be fasting that day. That's okay. Don't scratch the fast or beat yourself up because of a mess-up. Simply acknowledge where you misstepped, and dedicate the rest of your day to allowing God to refine you through the fasting process. Remember this isn't about flexing our spiritual muscles; it's about opening ourselves to the Spirit's refining work. Part of that is acknowledging that we desperately need Him, and that's a good thing.

This won't make much sense to the watching world, but to those of us who belong to God, we proclaim with each fast: "I live not by bread alone (or chocolate, or ice cream, or my skinny dolce latte) but by You, Lord. And even if I never again taste my favorite treat, I will be happy and fulfilled in You!"

David Mathis explains, "We fast from what we can see and taste because we have tasted and seen the goodness of the invisible and infinite God—and are desperately hungry for more of him."[5] The more we feast on God, the more we will desire to fast from the gifts that seduce our souls so that we may turn our hearts back to Him. Our appetites for God will be awakened, and we'll find that His presence sustains us whatever we face.

Jesus can handle our emotional highs and lows, giving us grace and mercy, joy and strength, and best of all, the pleasure of His own presence—things that can never be found in a candy bar.

Digest the Truth

(*for individual or group response*)

1. Have you ever fasted from food for spiritual reasons? What was your experience like?

2. In what way(s) has food become the focus of your attention instead of the way to direct your attention to the Giver?

3. Have you experienced God's ability to sustain you when stripped of other crutches like comfort foods? In what way have you used food to substitute what only God can provide?

4. Describe one experience in which you've tasted God's goodness personally.

Bonus Online Content

Download "The Full Life Bible Reading Plan" at http://www.thefull.life/reading-plan.

Jennifer's story

My love affair with food began in my teens. I was pursuing a professional career as a dancer and being underweight was the goal. I spent equal time obsessing over my measurements to obsessing over my next binge. It was a slow realization that I ate when I was way past full and that I was no longer listening to my body or the Lord but rather to this slave driver named "fill me"!

It's been a grace work of God over the last twenty years, in increasing measure setting me free. We all turn to something to fill us, to make us feel better. God in His grace causes us to open our blind eyes, pull us off the path of lambs to the slaughter for that next binge, and come to Him to be truly satisfied.

I have days of amazing victory where I silence my flesh and feast on the Lord, His word, Himself. The apostle Peter says it's like being a baby on the breast hungrily devouring the Word of God because we know it's good for us; it will make us grow and mature. I praise God for those days, and in increasing measure they are more than my days of failure and giving in to the lust of my flesh and overeating.

Praise God I no longer am a slave to my measurements. He broke that chain, and by His grace He will keep me in the center of His will which is a place of moderation, balance, sanity, and freedom!

6

Feast on God's Word

My husband and I recently shared a slice of chocolate fudge cake with chocolate syrup and ice cream.

If you think that sounds decadent, you're right. It was.

With each forkful, my taste buds exploded with pleasure, sending rapid signals to my brain saying, "Get a load of this!" I savored each morsel, telling myself that I would stop with that bite. But a few seconds later, I reached for another. *Just one more bite*, I promised myself, as Flaviu and I passed the fork back and forth.

Chocolate is addictive that way. It seems to satisfy in the moment, but it makes you crave just a little more.

While an addiction to chocolate leads to terrible health complications, an addiction to God's Word leads to spiritual wholeness. And if we take the psalmist's word for it, God's

Word is just as sweet and satisfying: "How sweet are your words to my taste, sweeter than honey to my mouth!" (Psalm 119:103).

I'm not a big fan of honey, so this verse never meant much to me. But when I substituted the word "brownies" for honey . . . well, suddenly this verse took on a whole new meaning: Those who enjoy God's presence feast on His Word as if it was the tastiest treat in the world.

But the problem is that for most of us, God's Word doesn't sound nearly as appealing as a chocolate milkshake. After all, when's the last time you were driving your car around town and thought, *Mmm . . . I'm really craving the Bible. I think I'm going to pull into a parking lot and read a few verses to meditate on my way home.* Sounds a bit silly, doesn't it? But Scripture tells us that those who have tasted the richness of God as revealed in His Word can't get enough of Him, much like a chocolate addict can't stop with just one bite of cake.

Psalm 119 is the longest chapter in the Bible, dedicated entirely to praising the goodness of God's Word. Of the 176 verses in the chapter, all but five mention God's Word, His promises, His commands, or His precepts. The psalmist was definitely enamored with God and what He had to say because he discovered that nothing satisfies more than God Himself.

Just look at some of the ways he describes it in this chapter alone. God's Word:

Brings blessings to those who follow it (v. 2)

Protects the reader from sinning against God (v. 11)

Causes as much celebration as winning the jackpot (v. 14)

Revives a weary and burned-out soul (v. 25)

Brings freedom and liberty (v. 45)

Brings assurance of God's promises (v. 58)

Is more delightful than artery-clogging delicacies (v. 70)

Is consistent throughout millennia and all over the world (v. 89)

Provides direction in life (v. 105)

Delights the believer even in the midst of heartache (v. 143)

Gives us a vocabulary to praise God when we don't know what to say (v. 171)

The psalmist discovered so much richness in God's Word, and that's just summarizing eleven of the 176 verses in the chapter! Can you imagine how full his heart must have been to have it flow over into pages and pages of declarations of love? This writer had experienced firsthand the richness of God's Word in his own life, both in good seasons and in hard ones, and he eagerly desired others to discover the same lasting comfort in God as he did.

Through his lifelong study and devotion to God's law, the psalmist discovered that nothing satisfies quite like God Himself. Jim Cymbala explains this connection: "When we eat a good meal, we forget about it in twenty-four hours; but when the Lord feeds us his Word, we have food for our souls that lasts forever."[1] That food that nourishes our inner person continues to feed us even months or years after we first read it, and the deeper we dig into His Word, the more satisfied we become.

And while most of us won't go on to write an award-winning tome about God's Word, we too can discover the abundance of riches that are ours in the Bible. When we learn to feast on God's Word through study, memorization, and meditation, we will come to know and love God more, finding a real and lasting satisfaction in Him that helps us set aside our food fixation.

With Heart and Mind

For too many years, I read the Bible to learn more about myself: how I should live, what I should do, who I am in Christ, what sort of spiritual heritage I have from all the heroes of the Bible. Maybe you've done that too. And there's plenty of that in the Bible.

But that's not the main point.

If we read the Bible to come up with a list of rules for how to live, we're going to miss the most incredible story of love and redemption this earth has ever seen.

The Bible isn't about us. The Bible is about God.

Throughout Scripture, God reveals Himself to us in beautiful stories of personal redemption. These themes repeat again and again—how God is faithful even when His people are not, how He provides for His children though a situation looks dire, and how He keeps working humans' good toward His glory. It's an incredible story that's drama, suspense, comedy, thriller, and romance all in one.

And this story is all about God. If we read it any other way, we'll get bored fast.

In our journey toward healthy eating, we study the Bible not to uncover a secret path to victory but to better know God. He is our victory. He is our prize.

So we read the Bible to learn about God.

But it's not enough to know more about God if our minds don't affect our hearts. Our study of God must lead us deeper in love with God too. Because unless all this information results in God-adoration, reading the Bible is pointless.

Our Bible study each day should culminate not in a list of things to do but in a million reasons to worship. Bible study and worship go hand in hand, like peanut butter and jelly, salt and pepper, and every other pair you can think of, but better. We can't have one without the other if we really want to grow in our relationship with God.

Here's what happens when we have worship without study: Some people want to love God, but they don't really know Him. God is a caricature of all the stories they've heard in Sunday school, a one-dimensional figure resembling either jovial Santa Claus or moody Zeus. They don't quite know how to reconcile God's love *and* justice, His mercy *and* holiness, His omniscience *and* His gift of free will. They are all love and little knowledge.

Then again, there's the other extreme of study without worship: Other people know much about God, but there's little about Him that moves them. They can expound on atonement and transubstantiation in one breath and in the next yell at the driver who cut in front of them in traffic. Simply put, their knowledge of God is merely a cerebral endeavor; it hasn't affected their posture toward the one they have learned about. God is something to be analyzed and dissected, not someone to worship and adore. They are all knowledge and little love.

But we are called to love God with both our hearts *and* our minds: "Love the Lord your God with all your heart and with all your soul and with all your mind and with all your strength" (Mark 12:30).

"The heart cannot love what the mind does not know."[2] In studying Scripture, we can know God better and love Him more deeply. In fact, this is the point of reading the Bible, not to grow in head knowledge of biblical facts but to grow in our love and admiration of our Savior. Bible study must drive us to God in worship. Head knowledge without love is useless (see 1 Corinthians 13:1–3). This central truth was pivotal in my journey toward finding joy in Scripture again: As I grow in knowledge and worship of God, I will grow deeper in my love for Him too. And the more we love Him, the more we will worship and glorify Him, whether we're reading a devotional, folding laundry, sweeping the floor, or eating a brownie.

Because, yes, you can eat a brownie for God's glory.

How to Feast on God's Word

He was famished.

Starving, really. Having spent forty days and nights in the desert fasting and praying, and being tempted by Satan (Matthew 4:1–11), Jesus faced the devil's offer to turn stones into bread.

Yet He refused to be distracted by Satan's tricks: "Jesus answered, 'It is written, "Man shall not live by bread alone, but by every word that comes from the mouth of God"'" (v. 4).

"Every word that comes from the mouth of God" refers to God's self-revelation, and we get these words of revelation most obviously through studying Scripture. But in our journey toward healthy eating, we study the Bible not to uncover a secret path to victory but to better know God. He is our victory. He is our prize. We look for Him on every page and we run to Him with every verse. Our hearts cry out for more of Him in our lives.

So how do we do this, practically?

Go with Anticipation

Jesus knew that there is more to life than what we eat and drink. God, not food, is the source of our life; it is on Him alone that we depend.

In our journey toward overcoming food fixation, we must continually reset our hearts and minds to this default truth: we live for God, not for the next meal. He is our reward. His presence is more comforting than anything we put in our mouths. We experience abundant life when we hang on God's every word rather than think about what's for dinner.

Practically speaking, we must ask ourselves: "What do I desire more—God's presence or food?" If the answer is not in line with Jesus' answer to Satan, then we must pray for God to change our hearts, and keep praying until we experience change.

Regardless of your current appetite for Scripture, ask God to develop in you a hunger for His Word, and then set aside a regular time to feed your soul. Leland Wang, a Chinese minister who helped spark an evangelical revival in China in the early 1900s, revealed his simple plan for systematic Bible study: "No Bible, no breakfast."[3] He decided to read a portion of Scripture each day before allowing food to pass his lips, and his grumbling stomach provided incentive enough to open his Bible. My own father followed a similar pattern, and I have fond memories of watching him sit at the breakfast table (though it was often more like brunch or lunch as he is a late riser), to read even just a verse before digging into my mom's delicious cooking.

The point is not to become legalistic in checking something off our spiritual to-do list but rather to develop habits that will encourage our pursuit of God in a world rife with distractions.

Just Get Started

We are so fortunate to live in a time and place where God's written Word is readily available to us in print, online, and through many smartphone apps. Unfortunately, we rarely take advantage of this blessing. If you want to hunger for God, you need to know His Word, and the easiest way to do that is to study what He's already revealed to us as recorded in the Bible.

We might think we don't have time, but the truth is we all have the same twenty-four hours in our day—we must simply choose what we do with it. Start reading a few verses a day, and share what you're learning. As His Word comes alive to you, I promise you'll get excited to dig deeper into it, because you'll see God on every page and run to Him with every verse.

Use a Simple Method

Whether you're new to Bible study or have been studying the Bible for many years, this FEAST method will bring richness to your personal quiet time and increase your love and knowledge of God.[4]

Focus

Ask the Spirit of God to focus your heart and mind on Him. Then choose a passage to focus on during your study time.

Engage

Read the passage and engage it by writing down observations (who, what, when, where, why, how). Be careful to use "them," "there," and "then" language when answering the question, "What does it say?"

Assess

Consider the context and genre of the passage as well as the cultural and historical background by checking cross-references and commentaries. Assess the main idea of the passage by answering the question, "What did it mean to the original audience?"

Spark

Ask the Holy Spirit to spark transformation in your life by applying the passage in specific and measurable ways. Ask "How can I apply this?" and prayerfully commit to one small action that immediately implements what you learned.

Turn

As you end your study of Scripture, turn your mind and heart toward God in worship. Respond to Him with praise, confession, and thanksgiving.

Whatever method you use to study the Bible, take time each day to chew on a few verses. There are few things more exhilarating than feeling God speak directly to a situation in your life right now through words that were penned thousands of years ago. His Word is living and active. Experience it for yourself, and you'll understand what Jesus meant when He said we live by God's Word, not by food.

Memorize—Yes You Can!

As we study God's Word, specific verses will strike us to the heart, and we think, *I really want to remember that.* And as we discussed in chapter 3, when we memorize God's Word, the Spirit of God brings those verses to mind when we need them most. Remember that the Sword of the Spirit, God's Word, is what we use to ward off temptation, but that's rather difficult to do when we don't have it handy. That's why we're called to hide God's Word in our hearts (Psalm 119:11).

Before you think, *Oh, I could never memorize Bible verses! I have a terrible memory!* let me assure you that I do too. In fact, I used that excuse for many years of my adult life, until one day I was helping my toddler learn a Bible verse for her Sunday school class, and I memorized it with her! This phenomenon happened the next week, and the next, and the next, until I realized my problem wasn't that I couldn't memorize Scripture— my problem was that I hadn't intentionally pursued memorizing Scripture.

Memorizing Scripture takes effort and intentionality, but it's neither impossible nor is it a waste of time.[5] The trick is to select passages that have meaning and relevance to what you're facing at the time. If you're in a battle to overcome food fixation, then arm yourself with the Sword of the Spirit by memorizing Scriptures that speak to that particular stronghold. Then use temptations as opportunities to recall those verses to mind and use them to speak God's truth into your life, much like Jesus did in His wilderness temptations.

No one ever taught me how to memorize Scripture, so in my "I-can't-memorize" days, I would sit down with a verse and repeat the whole verse over and over again, growing frustrated with my inability to recite it back after ten sets of repetition. Perhaps you've experienced similar frustration.

But when I began memorizing Bible verses with my toddler, I went about it entirely differently. I divided the verses into short phrases. I used silly hand motions, and even tried singing a little tune. I would say a part and she would say it back to me, and pretty soon I found that neither of us needed promptings as we had quickly committed the verse to memory. Potty-training time became our Bible verse time, and over the course of a few weeks she learned two valuable skills, and I had discovered my memory wasn't as bad as I thought it was.

If you find it hard to remember Bible verses, here are some techniques I tried both with my toddler and by myself that have been wildly successful:

> Read the verse out loud several times, so you familiarize yourself with the words.

> Use hand motions that will remind you what phrase comes next.

> Repeat the verse several days in a row, so it moves into your long-term memory.

> Study the Bible verse, so you have a deep understanding of it.

Write verses on notecards and carry them in
your purse or wallet.

Put sticky notes above the sink to fill your
mind with truth while washing dishes.

Use a smartphone app to review memory
verses while waiting in the grocery line.

Listen to songs that are Scripture set to music.

Try to memorize Scripture that pertains to your current situation, and you'll be more likely to remember it when you need to wield that sword of the Spirit, either to ward off the midday munchies, fill you with joy, or remind you of eternal truth. If you're looking for specific verses to memorize in your journey toward food freedom, you'll find a list of the verses I memorized throughout my sugar fast toward the back of the book.

As we commit God's Word to memory, our cravings can become triggers to remind us to meditate on Scripture and be transformed into the image of Jesus Christ. And as we meditate on those verses, the Spirit brings the words to life as He applies them in our current situation.

Be Attuned to the Spirit

Those who have committed their lives to Jesus receive an amazing gift: the Holy Spirit of God, our Comforter. God also speaks through His Spirit who lives in us, inviting us to depend on Him at every turn.

At first, it may be difficult to quiet our spirits and listen to Him, but as we practice this discipline of stillness, we will begin to hear Him speak to us, first in a quiet whisper and then louder and more clearly as we obey.

The Spirit convicts us when we flirt with temptation, and He comforts us when we bring our brokenness to Him. Many times I'd open the cupboards to look for a snack, only to hear His voice gently asking me, *Why are you looking for comfort in what doesn't satisfy? Come to Me instead.* And every time I obeyed, He satisfied me with Himself. Only later did I realize those were verses from Isaiah that I had memorized weeks beforehand, coming back to memory at just the time I needed them, applied directly to my life. This is often how the Spirit works, bringing the Word to mind and guiding us into the way of life.

The truth is that God's Word is always applicable in our lives. Whatever we're facing, there's something in His Word that addresses it:

If you are impatient, sit down quietly and commune with Job. If you are strong-headed, read of Moses and Peter. If you are weak-kneed, look at Elijah. If there is no song in your heart, listen to David sing. If you are a politician, read Daniel. If you are getting sordid, read Isaiah. If your heart is chilly, read of the beloved disciple, John. If your faith is low, read Paul. If you are getting lazy, watch James. If you are losing sight of the future, read in Revelation of the promised land. In joy and sorrow, in health and in sickness, in poverty and in riches, in every condition of life, God has [something] stored up in His Word for you.[6]

Saturate yourself with Scripture so that when temptation hits, you're ready to fight back. And as you do this, you'll begin to discover an appetite for His Word you never thought you'd have.

As we feast on God's Word through these practices, we'll begin to discover the God of the Scriptures in a personal and intimate way. We will be full of His Word and His presence and will gradually cease craving cheap fill-ins. We begin to experience the sufficiency of God Himself, as we turn to Him and food fades into its proper place.

Digest the Truth
(*for individual or group response*)

1. Describe the power of feasting on God's Word. Have you ever experienced this? Have you tried to use God's Word to overcome temptation? What happened?

2. What steps are most important for wielding the Word of God as a sword?

3. In what ways have you found satisfaction in God so far? How can you use your experiences to encourage someone else on this journey?

4. How can you recognize when the Holy Spirit is giving you a message? In what ways can you "listen" to His voice and follow through?

Bonus Online Content
Download the FEAST bookmark for use in your personal Bible study at http://www.thefull.life/feast-bookmark.

Jenn's story

I'm thirty-five, a wife, and mother of four boys. Over the years I've been in and out of therapy sessions and eating disorder clinics for compulsive overeating. My struggle with food started when I was six years old, having been subjected to a very traumatic experience. I didn't tell my mom or anyone what had happened for fear that I would be in trouble or someone would get hurt, so I stuffed it all inside with food.

Food was the one thing I could control for myself, and the good feelings I received while eating sweets was a way of self-medicating the pain I was going through. It was almost a year before I told my mom about that terrible experience, and then I went through therapy, which helped some, though not a hundred percent.

During most of my childhood, people focused on my weight and how to help me lose the fat, but no one really stopped to wonder what was going on inside that made me want to eat like I had a bottomless hole, a hole nothing on earth could fill. At age seventeen, I became sexually active and sought for love in all the wrong places; I started using drugs recreationally. I was reckless and out of control, and for a long time I used sex and drugs as a way to fill the void I had instead of food. When I was twenty-two I hit rock bottom, and after such a stubborn road of trying to control everything and heal my own hurts, I turned to the Lord. I gave my life back to Him.

Over time, I've learned to actually feel my emotions, rather than stuff them down, and allow myself to process them. I keep a prayer journal and write out my emotions, thoughts, and anything going on in my life that's driving me to food. I still struggle with my relationship with food but I'm learning day by day to go to Jesus with my hurt instead of the brownies. Only He fills me with joy and sustains me more than any food on this earth can.

Part Three

Experiencing
Everyday Fullness

7

Discover
Your Triggers

Whenever I walk into my mom's kitchen, I look for something to munch on. It doesn't matter if I've just had lunch—just stepping foot into the kitchen is enough to make me start searching the table, countertop, fridge, and cupboards for something yummy. I guess you could say I've been trained to do so because my mom usually has something delicious on hand to feed us.

And really, who can say no to freshly baked apple strudel? Or made-from-scratch *placinta* (Romanian cheese-stuffed fried dough rounds)? Or any other scrumptious concoction she's got on hand? After all, I spent nearly twenty years cooking at her side, eating at her table, and sampling her latest creations. Like Pavlov's dog and the bell, I walk into her house and feel my mouth water with eager anticipation. And unfortunately,

I check all reason and self-control at the door. For as much as I love my mom's kitchen, it's become one of the places where I need to be most on guard, because the temptation to eat out of boredom, habit, or anxiety is overpowering.

Do you ever overstep your food boundaries at the same time of day or around the same people? That's an example of a food trigger, and—though you've already experienced victory—it can cause a return to former food fixation habits, like overeating, counting calories, and obsessing about every bite.

It's useful for us to determine what our particular triggers are, and when faced with that trigger, we can make the intentional choice of whether to go to God or go to food. In this chapter, we'll talk about the cycle, triggers, and how we can replace the spiral of temporary fixes with the lasting satisfaction found in Christ.

Trigger Warnings

Here are some common food fixation triggers.[1] You may resonate with many of these, and you can add your own.

> **Food triggers:** the smell of food cooking; seeing food in the bakery window, buffet, or fridge; vending machines filled with junk food; favorite comfort foods at a family gathering; any favorite foods (mostly carbs).
>
> **Behavioral triggers:** passive activities such as watching TV, working on the computer, or

reading a magazine; driving in the car; going to a party; eating out of habit; walking into the kitchen; not sleeping; procrastination.

Emotional triggers: anger, family interaction, low self-esteem, performance anxiety, feeling like "I deserve this," depression.

Environmental triggers: cultural expectations, eating with certain people, seeing a TV commercial featuring food, seeing a recipe or food advertisement, being out in cold weather, office coworkers bringing goodies to share or sell, time of day, going out to eat.

If you find yourself returning to former food fixation habits, it's a good idea to keep a log of triggers to help you identify which ones you're most susceptible to and come up with solutions to overcome them. For me, that means keeping a glass of water within reach whenever I'm at my mom's house and sipping that instead of constantly reaching for something to munch on.

The trigger itself isn't bad, but it can derail our efforts to find fullness in God by lulling us into old habits. When facing one of these situations, we have the choice to either turn to food or cry out to God to fill us instead.

Fleeing from the Idol of Comfort Food

One of the key verses for any person who's trying to resist temptation reads like this, "No temptation has overtaken you except what is common to mankind." You know it, right? It's a feel-good verse that gives us courage and hope as we face our own giants of temptation.

But the passage doesn't stop there. It goes on to say, "And God is faithful; he will not let you be tempted beyond what you can bear. But when you are tempted, he will also provide a way out so that you can endure it. Therefore, my dear friends, flee from idolatry" (1 Corinthians 10:13–14). How interesting that this passage about resisting temptation is followed so closely with an admonition to stay away from idolatry!

As we've discussed, whenever we turn to food to soothe us rather than going to God with our problems, we're essentially making food our idol. It's what happens if we drink a can of soda to fix our restless night or turn to the secret stash of chocolates when we get frustrated with the kids or mindlessly munch on crackers at the holiday party because we feel lonely or drown our sorrow of a botched date in a bottle of wine or a pint of ice cream.

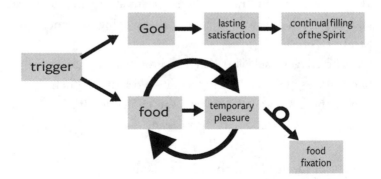

Whenever we eat to solve our emotional issues, we only exacerbate our problems, because once the initial pleasure of eating wears off, we feel guilt, shame, and disappointment in addition to the initial emotion that drove us to food in the first place. Food can't help us out; only God can.

With each bite, with each diet, with each newly discovered health craze, we're tightening the noose around our necks that suffocates the air out of our lives. Food obsession overwhelms us, but we don't know where else to turn. Until we turn away from our idols of food, health, skinny thighs, or whatever else we're trusting for our satisfaction, and turn instead to the one true God, we will never find freedom because "where the Spirit of the Lord is, there is freedom" (2 Corinthians 3:17).

Sadly, emotional eating is one of the most common manifestations of food fixation. It's easy to run to food for comfort instead of facing our emotions, especially when they're painful. The next time you're tempted to turn to food for comfort, prayerfully journal through these questions:

What's going on in my life right now that's making me want to eat?

What emotion am I experiencing?

Will eating make me feel better? If so, for how long?

Will eating solve my problems?

Will eating create any new problems?

What do my boundaries protect me from?

Do I need protection today?

What do I think God wants to teach me through this trial?

What can I thank God for in this situation?[2]

When we recognize that God is not only big enough to handle our problems but that He is the *only one* who can set us free, we properly acknowledge Him as the source of our satisfaction and we release food to its proper place: a good gift to be enjoyed from a good God.

Moses prayed, "Satisfy us in the morning with your unfailing love, that we may sing for joy and be glad all our days" (Psalm 90:14). If, like Moses, we turn to God each morning and ask Him to fill us with Himself, then we won't turn to food to meet those holes. When we're experiencing anxiety over a situation at work, we will more easily turn to God and ask His love to meet that need rather than brood over a plate of chocolate chip cookies. And when we hear good news, we will run straight to God, singing His praises for His provision.

Food simply loses its stronghold when there's no place for it to set foot. If all our needs are met in God, if He becomes our satisfaction every morning, then we can "sing for joy and be glad" all our days. No self-administered chocolate treatment required.

Because let's face it: food may provide a temporary relief from whatever situation or emotion presses in on us, but it's short-lived and soon replaced by feelings of guilt and despair. But God's love is everlasting. It's wider and longer and higher and deeper than what we can fathom (Ephesians 3:18). We can dive headfirst into His love and soak it in, enjoying it completely without worrying about unfavorable side effects. No added pounds. No stomach aches. No social stigma. Just pure, wonderful, abounding love and satisfaction.

Fleeing from the Idol of Self-Will

My natural recourse when I'm tempted again to turn to food is to buckle down and impose more rules on myself: "No more carbs. Only salads for lunch. No more desserts. Go running every day."

But truly, this approach has never lasted, because it's rooted in my own power and self-discipline, which as we've already established is severely limited and (ironically) leads to more legalism. Like Paul, I find myself bemoaning my lack of self-control. Anyone who has experienced weight gain due to food addiction can identify with these verses:

> I have the desire to do what is good, but I cannot carry it out. For I do not do the good I want to do [that is, eat small portions, choose healthy options, stop when I'm full and seek comfort in God, not food], but the evil I do not want to do [overeating, mindless bingeing, eating junk food, choosing immediate, temporal satisfaction in my next bite, midnight pantry raids]—this I keep on doing. Now if I do what I do not want to do, it is no longer I who do it, but it is sin living in me that does it. . . . Who will rescue me from this body of death? [And here is where desperation sets in, and so the resolve to start a new diet or the retreat to another box of cookies.] Thanks be to God, who delivers me through Jesus Christ our Lord. (Romans 7:18–19, 24–25)

Then in Romans 8, Paul provides insight into what life through the Spirit looks like:

The Spirit sets us free from the power of sin and death (vv. 1–4).

We are to become experientially what we already are positionally (vv. 5–10; see also Romans 6).

The Spirit empowers us to live as we could not on our own (vv. 11–16, 26–27).

Our present obedience and discipline prepares us for future glory (vv. 17–25).

As we live by the Spirit, our victory is secured, not just overcoming sin but being transformed into the image of Christ and experiencing deeper intimacy with God (vv. 26–39).

How is this "life by the Spirit" possible, if not by spending time in His presence, being conformed into the image of the Son (v. 29), as we gaze upon His beauty in admiration, bow our lives and will before Him in worship, and follow His example in discipline? Bill Hull says, "True conversion means discipleship, and further, that discipleship means discipline. We can experience great freedom when life's appetites serve God's kingdom rather than dominate our own lives."[3]

Our souls are wooed from the empty pleasures of this world when they experience greater satisfaction in the presence of God. And while that process may sometimes be pleasant, it is often painful, as we learn to say no to our selfish appetites (denying self and its demands as we follow the way of the cross), and yes to the Spirit (often the harder path, which reveals just how desperately we need God's grace).

If we were able to simply will ourselves to be more disciplined, that would not be mortification of the self; it would be exaltation of the self. This is why we sometimes see people who are extremely disciplined in some areas of their lives yet who are still far from God. The goal of overcoming food fixation is not to lose weight—it is to bring glory to God through our transformation into the image of the Son as we find complete joy and satisfaction in God.

We must die to ourselves, reaching the end of our own self-discipline and throwing ourselves on the mercies of God. Only then can the Spirit fill us with fresh power as He powerfully works through us to change our habits, appetites, and desires through the daily discipline of choosing God over food.

Let us posture ourselves in a position to receive the Spirit's infilling: eager, expectant, and earnest in worship.

Learning to Worship God

We can see the direct correlation between worship and discipline. The discipline of worship is daily coming before God and admitting: *You are enough. I need You.*

Like breathing in and out, this prayer rises within our hearts in an endless loop.

Breathe in. *I need You.*

Breathe out. *You are enough.*

This refrain is the cry of the psalms. This is the experience of the godly. This is the act of worship. Idolatry is the opposite: believing God is not enough and that I need something other than Him to be satisfied. When I'm not worshiping God, I'm worshiping something else. We humans were created to worship.

It's knit into our very beings. We cannot help it. We cannot *not* worship. But we *can* choose what—and who—we will worship, and all of Scripture is a call to worship the only one who is worthy: Jesus Christ, our Lord.

If we are to be completely satisfied with God, we need to experience Him for ourselves personally in all the nitty-gritty details of life.

And He invites us to experience His goodness personally, in our own lives, in the very places we hurt the most.

Imagine visiting the restaurant of a world-renowned chef. He walks into the dining room and invites you to come and watch him work in his kitchen. He's preparing his signature dish, and he wants you to see the whole process. You watch as he chops onions, carrots, celery, garlic, and red bell peppers, marveling at his swift movements. You hear the sizzle as he sears the beef and laugh along to his easy banter. You sniff the wafting aromas as he stirs the pot. You salivate as he ladles the concoction into a porcelain bowl, and when you taste his world-famous Bavarian beef stew, you experience for yourself the very reason this chef has gained his fame. The man can cook.

But getting to step behind the scenes and watch this masterful chef at work makes this meal even more special than if you had simply eaten it in the dining area. You watched the careful attention that went into preparing the dish, and you formed a connection with the chef. You gained a greater appreciation for him. Admiration even.

So it is with God. He invites us into His presence, not just to enjoy the blessings of a full life but to share the experience with Him, growing deeper in our love and admiration of Him. If we are to be completely satisfied with God, we need to begin recognizing Him in all the nitty-gritty details of daily life. It's one thing to acknowledge God's power over the whole world; it's an entirely different thing to celebrate His involvement in the details of your own life.

David understood this difference, and after listing the ways God answered his cries for help and protected him from danger, he in turn invites us to "taste and see that the Lord is good" (Psalm 34:8). It's like he's saying, "Don't take my word for it. Try Him for yourself!"

Notice that this taste test isn't to decide *if* the Lord is good; His goodness is an established reality. Our tasting simply introduces us to the pleasure of His presence, awakening our spiritual senses to marvel and wonder at His goodness.

Linda Dillow writes of this very concept in her moving book *Satisfy My Thirsty Soul*:

> I wanted more of God. I longed for a personal encounter with Him. God spoke to me in His Word, but I desired to hear His personal voice to me. I yearned for joy unspeakable, for a deeper union and oneness, for spiritual, bridal union. I didn't want to settle for God's omnipresence, where I knew He was everywhere, or even for His wonderful, abiding presence. I thirsted for a face-to-face intimacy with God.[4]

Later in the book Linda explains how the Holy Spirit changed her thinking and her life, growing in her a longing and adoration for God. As she learned to worship God, she found everything she was searching for—and more. So it was in my life. Linda's book was the spark God used to stir my heart with longings for Him, and gradually I began to taste His goodness for myself.

Let us not content ourselves with merely watching what God's doing in other people's lives. Let's not just listen to inspiring stories or read good books. Let us go all in. Taste and see that He *is* good. Extremely good. Amazingly good. So good, in fact, that all the other pleasures we've been running to pale in comparison to Him.

Satisfied with the Bread of Life

Jesus invites all who are thirsty to come to Him and find refreshment for our souls (Isaiah 55:1–2; John 4:14), a satisfaction that does not dwindle with time but only grows stronger as "rivers of living water will flow from within" (John 7:37–38), which is the Spirit who continually fills us up. Everything we need, we can find in Jesus.

No matter what the deeper issue is that's pushing us to look for satisfaction in food, we need to stop in our tracks and take it to Jesus instead. Only He is our Bread of Life; He is the daily sustenance that will keep us full, never to hunger again.

Breathe in. *I need You.* Breathe out. *You are enough.*

An endless chorus of praise that fills our hearts with joy and gladness all day, every day.

Digest the Truth

(*for individual or group response*)

1. What does a healthy relationship to food look like in your life?

2. List the foods you are most likely to overeat. What memories do you associate with each of them? When and where are you most likely to overeat? What are your food fixation triggers?

3. When triggers and cravings strike, how can you remind yourself to seek God instead of turning to food?

4. What leads you to return to food for comfort even though you already know it doesn't solve your problems?

5. Journal your eating for three days. Don't alter—just write down every bite you eat. Also note what emotions you felt immediately before and after eating. Do you see any patterns or connections? What surprises you? What reaffirms things you already knew about yourself?

Bonus Online Content

Watch Asheritah share about the power of personal worship, and access her personal worship playlist at http://www.thefull.life/worship-playlist.

Sara's story

I'm a pastor's wife and mom to five kids. I've struggled with my weight since I was three years old. My family liked to celebrate by eating out and overeating at holidays and family get-togethers. Eating was just something we did, and overeating was culturally acceptable.

As I got older, I continued to seek comfort in food and gained more weight. I would go on different diets and lose weight only to return to my old eating habits. Food was always within reach and became an easy way to cover up my feelings, but those decisions were destructive to my health and self. My life was completely out of balance, and I was taking care of others but neglecting my own health and wellness. I developed thought patterns that were so deeply entrenched that I needed professional help to break those thinking habits.

About twelve years ago, I began seeing a professional counselor. Over time, we processed the underlying reasons I was turning to food for comfort and all the other ways I was neglecting to care for myself. I learned that God has compassion on us and that we need to be compassionate with ourselves too. I changed my thinking, my core beliefs about who I am, and my deepest realizations about the way God loves and accepts me, and over time I lost a hundred pounds.

My journey continues to this day, and I help other women discover who God created them to be as they shed old habits and adopt new mindsets filled with God's truth, because nothing on the outside will fix what is broken on the inside.

8

Celebrate
the Gift of Food

I stirred the boiling water into the red gelatin as I tried
to make small talk. My mom was hosting a Fourth of July party
and had asked me and a few of her friends to come over early
to get everything ready.

"So, you work for a doctor?" I began tentatively, working on
the little information my mom had given me about her friend.

"I used to awhile ago," she answered. "I stopped working
there because I couldn't handle it anymore."

"How so?" I asked, peering at the bottom of the glass bowl
to make sure all the granules had dissolved.

She hesitated. "He was kind of out there in the nutritional
world. I learned the health risks associated with all these foods,
so I stayed on a strict diet of raw veggies. Honestly, I'd hardly

eat anything all day. By the time I quit my job, I was almost anorexic because of information overload. It seemed like whatever I wanted to eat would somehow lead to cancer. Even my veggies had to be sourced locally and organically. It just got to be too much."

I nodded, knowing the feeling of analysis paralysis in my food choices. After all, I still felt overwhelmed sometimes by all the information available about the dangers of eating this or that. So I was surprised to discover the refreshingly simple but profound message Scripture gives us about food: food is a good gift given by a good Father.

You may be familiar with the verse "So whether you eat or drink or whatever you do, do it all for the glory of God" (1 Corinthians 10:31). But have you ever thought of what that looks like in day-to-day life and why it even matters?

The Westminster Catechism, a collection of questions and answers about the Christian faith, begins with this pair: "What is the chief end of man? The chief end of man is to glorify God, and to enjoy him forever."[1] To glorify is to represent something as admirable, so our food choices, as everything else about our lives, should glorify Him. Sounds like a tall order for a simple lunch, doesn't it? But as we go back to the beginning of time, we will discover practical ways to turn mealtimes into daily acts of celebration.

Accept Food as a Good Gift

We serve a creative God. He could have created all vegetation to look the same and all animals to move the same; earth could have looked like a first-grader's drawing, but instead it reveals the genius of a Master Artist's work of art. God delighted in the beauty and variety He created, and He invites us to delight in it as well.

Enjoying food is not a sin; it's part of the reason God gave humans the gift of food in the first place.

Think back to the garden of Eden. God purposefully fashioned Adam and Eve with the physical ability to eat and digest food, deriving both energy and enjoyment from that food. This wasn't necessary. He could have created us to get energy from the sun, like plants do, or to be able to get all we need from oxygen. But He chose to create us in a way that requires us to regularly nourish our bodies with food. The act of eating reminds us that we are dependent on something other than ourselves for our survival, and numerous times in Scripture God uses food as a word picture of our dependence on Him as well. But God didn't just give us food for mere survival. If that were the case, He could have created one species of plants that produced energy flakes to give us all we needed to survive.

In His immense creativity and love, God gave Adam and Eve food for enjoyment as well. He created a cornucopia of delicacies—luscious fruits, crisp vegetables, crunchy nuts, and leafy greens, all with a unique texture, flavor, and color combination. And to make sure they could enjoy the food He created, our Father gifted them (and us) with the miracle of taste buds: millions of tiny receptors that send messages of pleasure to our brain and make us close our eyes with delight when we bite into a juicy pear or taste the creaminess of an avocado. On top of that, He gave humans a sliver of His creativity and intelligence to combine and prepare ingredients in such a way that the aroma alone would make our mouths water in anticipation of a delicious meal.

Enjoying food is not a sin; it's part of the reason God gave humans the gift of food in the first place. We know that Adam and Eve's enjoyment of food was not an afterthought for God; it was one of the primary reasons He gave them food in the first place, and it would have caused them to respond to their Creator with grateful hearts.

We see this theme of food as a good gift continue after the fall as well. When Noah and his family disembarked into a refreshed world, God invited them to enjoy all the pleasures of His creation: "Everything that lives and moves about will be food for you. Just as I gave you the green plants, I now give you everything" (Genesis 9:3). Thus God opened for humans a whole realm of food possibilities, including meat from animals. But as with many things in this fallen world, what God intends to be a blessing can quickly become a burden when we allow others to shape our view of God's gift.

Because we live in an age of information overload, we're surrounded by so-called experts who are happy to tell us which foods will likely kill us. Depending on which "expert" you're following, you have probably heard that meat, carbs, and dairy will all kill you; but you'll find just as many "experts" on the other side telling you that not eating these types of foods will bring dreadful consequences as well.

It's tempting to vilify entire food groups. I've gone through stages of avoiding one food item or another, only to discover that whatever I do, I'm pretty much doomed to die. On more than one occasion, I've stared in the cupboards for five minutes wondering what in God's world to eat for breakfast. *Cereal? Nope, too much sugar. Eggs? No, had those yesterday and I need to watch my cholesterol. Fruit smoothie? Nah, not enough protein to start my day. Gah!!*

It's enough to make me wish God would have created us solar-powered or perhaps given us a magic pill to swallow every morning so I wouldn't face a veritable health crisis every time I fill up my plate.

In moments like these, remember that food is not the enemy. Food is a gift from a loving Father meant to point us toward Him in joyful worship each time we take a bite. However, I'm not advocating an anything-goes approach to eating. We need to be wise and discerning with what we put into our bodies and in what quantities, especially since we live in a society filled with artificial foods. I'm simply saying, let's step back and recognize food as it was originally intended to be.

Lemon-blueberry scones are not of the devil—they are of the Father, a way to reflect the image of God in our creative use of the ingredients He has given us. And, yes, I do believe cooking and baking can be an act of worship if we turn grateful hearts to our Provider who has given us this canvas and these media to combine in artful fashion.

God has not restricted or withheld any food group from us, but He does charge us to be careful *how* we eat, and we'll address that later in this chapter.

Bless the Food

As she folds her little hands and squeezes her eyes shut, I can't help but smile. Our toddler mimics what she sees her mommy and daddy doing, even if she doesn't yet understand the concept of "blessing our food."

But sometimes I wonder if *I* even understand what that means.

As I neared the end of my sugar fast, I stumbled upon this gem in one of Paul's last letters: "Everything God created is good, and nothing is to be rejected if it is received with thanksgiving, because it is consecrated by the word of God and prayer" (1 Timothy 4:4–5).

How exactly is food consecrated? I wondered. As I studied the phrases "word of God" and "prayer," I discovered the traditional interpretation of this passage: praying before meals allows believers to consecrate their food in a special way, turning an otherwise mundane activity into a riveting time of worship.

Over a hundred years ago, at least one church leader had harsh words for those who hurried through such prayers as if they were an obligation to get through instead of a sacred pause: "[Grace before meals] too often denigrates into a mere form of words—into lip service of the most heartless form—and is too often looked upon as a kind of religious charm."[2] He urged his parishioners to pray with an honest and open heart, giving thanks to God continually.

The Apostolic Constitutions give us this ancient prayer, almost wholly consisting of Scripture:

> Blessed art thou, O Lord who feedest me from my youth, who givest food to all flesh: Fill our hearts with joy and gladness, that we, having all sufficiency, may abound unto every good work in Christ Jesus our Lord,

through whom glory, honor, and might be to thee forever. Amen.[3]

While most of our prayers will not be that ornate, the moment is still a built-in opportunity for worship, a chance to reorient our hearts toward God and ask for fresh power to overcome old eating habits.

Think about what you say for your typical pre-meal prayer. Do you follow the same formula before every meal, perhaps something along the lines of "Thank You, God, for this day and for providing us this food. Please bless it to nourish our bodies. Amen"?

There's nothing wrong with this, but we can do so much more. Especially for those of us who struggle with portion control, praying before meals can allow us to put food in its proper place before we begin. Imagine what kind of transformation you'd experience if you viewed meal times as worship times, not just once a day but every time you put something in your mouth!

Every time you sit down to a meal, thank God not just for providing your food but also for being your source of satisfaction. Tell Him that you recognize that food is a good gift for you to enjoy, and that you want to use this meal as an opportunity to worship Him for the ways He takes care of you. Ask the Spirit to help you know when to stop eating. Put food in its proper place by exalting God to His proper place.

Don't waste your pre-meal prayer times on halfhearted or hurried formulas. Turn each mealtime into worship time, sending the heart, grateful and glad, to the Giver.

Listen to Our Divine Dietitian

I've often wished for a personal trainer to follow me everywhere I go so she could step in and course-correct on the spot instead of letting one decision become a downward spiral of bad choices. And then it occurred to me that God gave us just that when He placed His Holy Spirit inside us. Jesus told us that He would send His Spirit to remind us of all the things He taught, and we're also told that He convicts us of sin and righteousness, as well as intervening for us before the Father.

In short, the Holy Spirit is like our own personal divine dietitian. He knows what is best for us, and He works within us if we let Him. We have no power of restraint or self-control without God's Word made alive in us by His Holy Spirit. Indeed, Paul tells us that self-control, along with joy, peace, patience, and so many other virtues, is the fruit of the Spirit (Galatians 5:22–23). It's the result of the Spirit working in us and transforming us into the image of Jesus Christ.

We can learn to listen to the Spirit and allow Him to lead our food choices. Here are a few practical ways to do that:

SOS intervention

You hover over the ice cream carton, spoon in hand. *I've had enough for tonight*, you realize, and you're ready to step away. But before you do, you think, *That was so good. I'll just have a few more spoonfuls.* Right there, in the space between that thought and your next action, you've reached your moment of decision.

Before any binge there comes a moment when we realize, "I should just stop right now. I've had enough." That is the voice of wisdom, the Spirit of God giving us an opportunity to choose to grow in Christlikeness by practicing immediate obedience. King Solomon put it this way: "Where there is no revelation, people cast off restraint; but blessed is the one who heeds wisdom's instruction" (Proverbs 29:18). Without an intervention from the Spirit of God, we find it difficult to practice restraint; but each time He reveals personal direction for us, we must heed His instruction to be blessed.

Some Christians bemoan the Spirit's silence in their lives when they ask for direction in big decisions or answers to hard questions. But how can we hear His still, small voice in those things when we close our ears to the very clear instructions in what's right in front of us? How do we expect to hear God's voice in unclear situations when we ignore Him in the plainest matters, like His call to worship, His call to refrain from self-indulgence, and His call to put down the chips and Netflix and pick up His Word instead?

> *The Holy Spirit is like our own personal divine dietitian.*

I have often excused my inaction under the guise of rejecting legalism—"I don't have to read the Bible to be close to God"—all while ignoring the blatant self-evident fact of the matter that what I'm currently indulging in doesn't bring me closer to God either and, in fact, I'm doing very little in such a season to pursue God. As I give in to my selfish nature, I crave even more things of my selfish nature. We crave what we consume.[4] So disobedience in one area of our lives often snowballs into other areas, until we're neither spending regular time in contemplative worship and confession nor are we eating from a place of satisfaction.

Instead, listen to the voice of God when He's calling you to obedience in the little things. Look for those moments of decision throughout your day. Listen for His promptings and obey immediately. You'll always be glad you did.

Food Rules

We've already established that food is a good gift, but we also need to guard against allowing any food to gain mastery over us. We each have our areas of weakness, so it's wise to invite the Spirit to help us establish our own food rules. What guidelines should we put up *for ourselves* to keep us from returning to food bondage?

A food choice may not be bad in itself, but we need to check if we're placing ourselves under the power of something or someone other than God. It is for freedom that Christ has set us free, and we need to constantly guard this freedom to keep from becoming enslaved to our appetites again.

One personal food rule that I observed for a long season of my recovery was that I only ate sweets with my husband, and even then only had one serving. This rule kept me from dangerous scenarios where I was tempted to return to old eating patterns, and often when I was tempted to forget it, the Spirit brought it to mind.

Your food rules will look different from mine, but prayerfully consider what guardrails you need to keep you on the narrow path. Some people avoid eating after 8:00 p.m.; others eat unprocessed foods during the week and enjoy a wider variety of foods on the weekends; others still eat whatever foods they want as long as they're homemade. The point here is not to return to an obsession with food rules, but rather to establish boundaries that will allow us to enjoy freely without constantly wondering what we can and cannot eat. As these food rules become habits, we will free up mental space and willpower to turn our attention outward.

Loving with Food

Look for ways to love others with food. Leave the last piece of peach crumble for your coworker. Give your friend the bigger half. Pick your spouse's favorite restaurant when going out to eat. Share those freshly made cookies with your church's pastoral staff instead of hoarding them at home.

Food has a way of making us turn inward and become selfish, but it can also be a powerful tool in God's hands if we let it. Ask the Spirit of God to transform food from a struggle into a mission field.

Eating to glorify God doesn't have to be a mystery—it's simply agreeing with God that food is a good gift, using mealtimes to reorient our hearts toward Him, and allowing His Spirit to personally guide us in freedom from our food struggles.

As we learn to listen to the Spirit's voice and obey His prodding, we will grow in discipline and control, mastering our bodies and cravings instead of allowing them to master us. And in that discipline, we will discover freedom that will last a lifetime.

Creating Healthy Eating Habits

For the longest time, I viewed discipline as a negative. But at the root of the word is *disciple*, a follower or apprentice, and that's a word that has a positive connotation. Discipline isn't just about being punished for doing something bad; discipline is about following the example of Jesus, living every second in line with this reality: God satisfies, and I need Him.

Discipline is like a muscle: it grows stronger the more we exercise it. The first time we say no to self and yes to the Spirit, it might feel impossibly hard. But the next time will be a bit easier, until obedience brings our spirit so closely in tune with God's Spirit in us that we don't have to wrestle over doing what He says. So the image of Christ is imprinted upon us, and we grow into maturity in Him.

In this aspect, our food choices can be viewed as a barometer of our spiritual growth and maturity. As we become more disciplined in our eating habits, we will find it easier to glorify God with our eating.

Habits can help us establish healthy eating patterns that train our hearts to seek God first. "God gave us habits so that we wouldn't have to find it necessary to keep relearning the common, mundane functions of our daily lives."[5] Imagine how draining and time-consuming it would be to have to think through the process of brushing your teeth each time or mentally listing the steps involved in driving a car. We would never have time or mental capacity to actually *do* anything of importance because all our energy would be drained by reviewing the basic necessities.

> *It is possible to break the cycle of a lifetime of dieting or calorie-counting or preoccupation with food or even an outright addiction.*

Habits are a beautiful gift that help us master a skill and then automate that process whenever we need it so we can focus on the more important things in life. Even better, we have the ability to learn new skills and create new habits as long as we live—it's never too late to start. So we *can* change, even if a learned behavior has been engraved into our lifestyle.

Remember, the Holy Spirit is able and willing to work powerfully in us to break us of our old nature and create in us the sanctified Christlike nature that honors God. The Spirit of the one who raised Jesus from the dead lives in us—can He not break our midnight snacking habit? We just need to consciously make the effort several times in a row, and eventually it will become easier and more natural, requiring less concentration and effort until it seems second nature.

Many of us have ingrained eating habits that are destructive to our health, whether that's the food choices we make, the size of our portions, or even the mental obsession. In fact, these habits can be so ingrained in us that we think we'll never be able to break them. But before you despair, remember that it *is* possible to break the cycle of a lifetime of dieting or years worth of meticulous calorie-counting or excessive preoccupation with food or even an outright addiction.

Yes, it will take time and discipline and it will be hard . . . but it can be done. In fact, the part of our brains that causes addictive behavior, like seeking cocaine, hitting the bottle, or diving into a bag of potato chips can be reprogrammed to once again function as God created it to.[6] Our habits are strong, but God promises to give us victory when we fight temptations: "Resist the devil, and he will flee from you" (James 4:7).

The New Testament does not provide a list of foods to eat and foods to avoid; for the believer, all foods are morally neutral. But it is our responsibility to be wise stewards of our bodies and make wise choices, and this includes avoiding foods that may harm our bodies. Does this mean I never eat a brownie again? Ultimately, that's between me and the Lord. I must not become enslaved, and I must care for my body.

Eating in a way that glorifies God, that points people to Jesus instead of drawing attention to our eating habits is a good thing. And because of this, I'm convinced that God will give us the knowledge, strength, and determination to make healthy choices. God wants us to experience freedom from food bondage even more than we do, so we can trust Him to complete the good work that He started in us and rejoice in His amazing love.

Digest the Truth
(*for individual or group response*)

1. In what ways have you been told that food is the enemy? Growing up, what was said (explicitly or implicitly) about the purpose of food? Was it accurate? How did that input influence the way you view food?

2. Why did God create food and taste buds? Does it make sense to you that "food is a gift from a loving Father meant to point us toward Him in joyful worship each time we take a bite"? How would your eating change if you adopted this view of food?

3. What does it mean to eat and drink to the glory of God (1 Corinthians 10:31)? What would this look like, practically, in your life? Are any foods inherently sinful or bad?

4. What does it mean to "bless this food," and how can praying before meals become a significant act of worship and a spiritual weapon?

Bonus Online Content

Download "The Blessing" printable for turning mealtime prayers into worship time at http://www.thefull.life/food-blessing.

Katie's story

After church I was grocery shopping and had an uncanny urge to indulge in some silky dark chocolate. At the time, I was taking a break from refined sugar, along with Asheritah and a large community of women, in order to crave Jesus and crush idols. I decided to investigate why I was experiencing such a ravenous craving. As I pushed my cart down the aisle, I threw the question up to the rafters. The Holy Spirit quickly unwrapped the core issue of my hungry heart.

At church that morning there were numerous issues that arose that were unexpected, difficult, and could not be controlled by my tightly wound self. Since I could not control other people or circumstances, I wanted to grab a treat to soothe my soul. It was a classic case of self-medicating in order to numb the symptoms of sin that were present. As this revelation came, I realized how often I reach for food in an effort to feel in control. I grab for a goodie when life is sweet and I sneak a snack when life is bitter. But I'm left feeling empty as I choose to partake in a temporary fix.

Deep within is a longing to be satisfied with Christ—for Him to be enough for me, for His daily bread to be sufficient instead of gorging on an excess portion of manna. Several years ago, I heard these words from Job 23:12: "I have not departed from the commands of his lips; I have treasured the words of his mouth more than my daily bread." I could not say this was true of me. I was treasuring my daily bread much more than the Bread of Heaven. It was time for a change, but it required laying down control in order to taste of God's goodness.

9

Run to Win

I'm a closet perfectionist. Seriously.

I stopped drawing in second grade because my drawings weren't as impressive as my friend's. For the longest time, I put off starting a blog because I didn't think anyone would read it. And for the first twenty years of my life, I told myself and others that I couldn't run, because I didn't sprint like a gazelle, as many of my friends did.

And even years into my marriage, I didn't make *sarmale*, my husband's favorite Romanian dish, because I didn't think I could live up to our mothers' renditions of it.

Basically, if I wasn't able to excel at something, I avoided doing it at all.

And for many years, this tactic worked. I focused on the things I was good at and avoided the things I was bad at. And in the process, I even managed to convince myself that I was an all-around disciplined person.

Then God drew my attention to my food addiction. And I realized that, try as I might, I just couldn't get a handle on the way I used and abused food. When Jesus finally set me free, I rejoiced, believing that I would now be released from all future struggles with food.

But that's not how the story goes.

The Myth of the Spotless Life

Even after I experienced God's divine intervention and the breaking of food's stronghold in my life, I continued to wrestle with food idolatry. I would swing wildly on the pendulum from "food is a necessary evil that I need to micromanage every second of my life" to "food is the best thing ever and if a little is good, then a lot is better." While I didn't return to a place of bondage, I continued to wrestle with moderation—aware of my decisions, eyes opened to God's power, and yet still choosing to sneak in an extra bite.

And honestly? This reality shocked me. How is it that one can experience God's divine power and intervention, and yet continue to struggle with the same thing over and over again? Why couldn't God dramatically intervene and give me victory for good? I wanted to be set free from addiction immediately and forever, but God often doesn't work that way.

God could fight [your addiction] all alone. He really doesn't need your help; however, God reserves the right to involve us in our own victories, so get ready to fight. Overcoming addiction may be the battle of your life. But it will also be the most rewarding, liberating victory of your life. It will be your own Goliath story for the rest of your days.[1]

For many of us who have grown up in church, we carry with us a heavy load of shame over our shortcomings.

God deserves our best, we were told; He will accept nothing less. So somewhere in the depths of my childhood psyche, the thought lodged in my mind that God wants me to be perfect.

And I tried. I tried really hard to be perfect. But time and time again I failed. Like the apostle Paul, no matter how hard I tried to do what was right, I kept doing what was wrong. Not only was I failing God but I felt I was also disappointing Him. Does any of this sound familiar to you?

I knew I couldn't be righteous on my own. I knew that I was born in sin and I needed God's grace to save me. I knew that Jesus died for my sins, and that He offered forgiveness freely and unconditionally to all who believe in Him.[2] But for some reason, I thought that once I was saved, I had to make God proud, to show Him He had chosen well to include me in His grace family.

It sounds kind of silly typing it out, but the struggle was real. And some days it still is. Having been justified by grace through faith, I thought I should be able to walk victoriously in perfection for the rest of my days.

When God the Father looks at me, He sees the perfect spotless Lamb of God. And if you're a believer in Jesus Christ, it's the same for you.

Because God wants us to be spotless, right? As spotless as the sacrificed lambs under the old Levitical law.[3]

All the while, I seemed to have forgotten that there is only *one* spotless One. Only *one* who lived a perfect life. God is not surprised by my failings. He is not taken aback when I eat a slice more of pizza than I should. He isn't *tsk-tsk*ing up in heaven over my lack of self-control. He does not reject me when I fail.

Do you know why?

Because when God the Father looks at me, He sees the perfect spotless Lamb of God. And if you're a believer in Jesus Christ, it's the same for you. Jesus died for your overeating, idolatry, gluttony, and every other sin you've ever committed in order to save you from eternal separation from God.

This is grace: not that we deserve God's approval but that it is given to us, transferred to us from the perfect Son of God to imperfect you and me. As Paul explains to the Roman church, "through the obedience of the one man [Jesus] the many will be made righteous" (Romans 5:19). Did you catch that? "Will be made." That's future tense. At the end of our lives, when we are united with Christ, we will be made perfect. But until then, we will continue contending with an imperfect body and an imperfect will in an imperfect world.

We cannot be spotless. And God doesn't expect us to be. There is only one Spotless One, and He offers to cover our imperfection with His perfect presence. Because of Jesus' spotless sacrifice for us, we are free to pursue victorious lives on our way to perfection in glory.

Five Principles for Lifelong Victory

1. Confess Your Continual Need for God

Humbly submit yourself and your problems to God, asking for His help and intervention. Recognize that any change needs to start with God, and you need His help. "Call on me in the day of trouble; I will deliver you, and you will honor me" (Psalm 50:15).

God is willing and able to help us, if only we would cry out to Him. This requires humility and intentionality—not just thinking about asking God for help but actually stopping in the middle of our distress and talking to Him.

One of the most effective tools I've discovered in overcoming food fixation is regular confession. We would do well to keep short accounts with God, not only confessing the ways we have failed Him daily but celebrating the ways He saves us. Honesty sometimes means keeping a food log so as to expose the hidden bites here and there. Honesty can also mean checking in with a friend to keep us accountable.

And honesty also looks like assessing reality as it truly is, free of deceit and untruthfulness, admitting when we've slipped, asking for help, and maintaining humility.

2. Seek Satisfaction in God Alone

Food fixation is not a new phenomenon; it's been around for thousands of years. In Philippians 3:18–19, Paul has strong words for those who are controlled by their appetites. He describes those whose "god is their stomach" as "enemies of the cross of Christ."

And so we once were, refusing to acknowledge what Jesus has done on the cross or to accept the freedom from sin that

He offers. We used to follow our cravings and passions, living self-centered and shallow lives. But not anymore! As we've surrendered our lives to God, we experience the power of Jesus Christ to break through our strongholds and set us free from our addiction to food.

And even as we begin to taste that freedom each day, we recognize that our bodies are still under the influence of our sinful nature. So, with Paul, "we eagerly await a Savior from [heaven], the Lord Jesus Christ, who, by the power that enables him to bring everything under his control, will transform our lowly bodies so that they will be like his glorious body" (Philippians 3:20–21).

We surrender our lives completely to Him, knowing that He has the power "to bring *everything under his control*" (3:21), even our intense cravings for food or our brain's chemical responses trained by years of indulging our sweet tooth. Someday we will be free of cravings that wage war with our good intentions. Our bodies will no longer fight against us but will be perfectly submitted as we go about doing the Lord's work.

3. Watch Expectantly for God's Deliverance

Once we admit we need God and ask Him to intervene, we need to believe He will do so.

This is where faith comes in. It's not enough to say a prayer and continue living as we did before. We must continue praying and believing, looking for God's deliverance and *expecting Him to change us.* For some, deliverance may be an overnight change, but for many others, it will take time. Watch and pray. God can free you if you cry out to Him and trust Him, and that often comes by giving us the power to resist the enemy. Even this is

God's provision and deliverance, even in the ordinary. Look for it, recognize it, and praise Him for it. As it says in Psalm 130:5–6:

> I wait for the Lord, my whole being waits,
>   and in his word I put my hope.
> I wait for the Lord
>   more than watchmen wait for the morning,
>   more than watchmen wait for the morning.

Be willing to wait as long as it takes. God isn't on the timetable we're on. We may want to look good for swimsuit season, but God has a bigger plan in mind. We must learn to trust and wait on Him. Like the persistent widow (Luke 18:1–5), we must continue to ask God to move in us, not because He is reluctant to, but because He often works through our continuous requests to create in us the desire needed to result in lifelong change. Wait as long as it takes, and in the meantime, do the next right thing (Isaiah 40:31).

4. Get Back Up

Let's face it: as we battle any stronghold, we will experience both victories and defeats. And relapsing into our previous behaviors is not uncommon.

When I experienced my first relapse into harmful food habits, I despaired. How could this happen when Jesus had set me free? Did running to the bag of chocolate chips after that argument invalidate the work I thought God had done in my life? Was it all in my head? Had I fallen from grace, never to get up?

If you've ever fallen off the wagon and just given up, I'm sure you can relate. Which is why it's so important for us to differentiate between the one-time work of Jesus and the ongoing work of sanctification. As Christine Caine writes, "Being set free and walking in freedom are not the same. The first was done for us by Jesus, but the second we must choose to do ourselves in His strength and by His grace."[4]

Some people may experience an immediate release from their addiction, but for the vast majority of us, victory comes as part of a journey made of small daily steps toward God. And that's okay, because God is more interested in teaching us to rely on Him in the journey than He is to speed us to our destination. His goal to refine us and mold us into the image of Jesus Christ takes time.

It's important to know how to handle our failures.

It's important, then, to know how to handle our failures. We must be quick to recognize our sin—which keeps us from hearing His voice and steals our joy—and to confess it to Him.

Sin and shame are two very different things. We can and must confess our sins. But we also must repudiate shame and condemnation—those never come from our Father but rather from the enemy, and they're intended to keep us hidden away from God, further distanced from Him.

When we experience a relapse or failure on our road to recovery, rather than wallow in our guilt or failures, we must rush to the cross of Jesus and confess our need for Him. God stands ready and willing to forgive us our sins and wipe the slate clean (1 John 1:9).

In other words, we must be honest. Both with ourselves and with God. Ask Him to show you where you went wrong, and what you need to do differently to continue walking in freedom and victory. Instead of allowing a mistake to send you into a tailspin, try one of these activities to get you back on track:

Talk to a close friend about what happened.

Journal through the emotional eating questions and the Evaluate Your Current Situation questions in chapter 12.

Describe the unmanageability this setback caused in your life.

Listen to the stories of others as a way to regain hope for change.

Ask God for help.

Accept the help and suggestions of those who are familiar with your story.

Call others who have struggled similarly— even just calling to say hi and leaving a short, encouraging message helps two people: It helps you get out of your obsessive thinking. And your encouraging words give someone else hope for change.

Forgive yourself.

Practice self-care: take a bath, read a book, take the dog for a walk.

Avoid triggering situations.

Ask for God's forgiveness.[5]

We surrender our bodies, minds, and spirits to God each day, disciplining our cravings and bringing them before the Lord. And as we do so, we're reminded just how much we need Him.

Remember, we're in this for the long run, not for the short win.

5. Celebrate Victories

We need to be both faithful and persistent in our prayers. Make focused prayer a priority each day, being confidently assured that what you're asking God for *will* become reality if it's in line with His will for your life.

As you pray, this hoped-for wish becomes reality, first in your heart and then in your life (Mark 11:23–24). Don't be discouraged by lack of progress or by doubters who scoff at your high hopes for change. Keep trusting that He who called you will continue to work in you. God loves us, and He will work in our lives as we persistently (Luke 11:5–8) ask Him to transform us into the image of His Son.

> Now to him who is able to do immeasurably more than all we ask or imagine, according to his power that is at work within us, to him be glory in the church and in Christ Jesus throughout all generations, for ever and ever! Amen. (Ephesians 3:20–21)

Wait for the Lord to act, and when He does, celebrate His victory!

As You Were Created to Live

Our mental energy was once preoccupied with food: dreaming of food, avoiding food, preparing food, looking up recipes on Pinterest, reading cookbooks, watching the Food Network.

But as God works in our lives, He frees us from food's controlling force, and we discover space within us that God wants to fill. Yes, with Himself first and foremost, but also with the purpose for which He created us. Too many Christians stifle their spiritual gifts and callings because they're too preoccupied with this food fixation. But as God frees you from that, you can begin discovering the purposes for which God created you in the first place.

You may already have a clear idea of God's purpose for your life, but if you don't, ask yourself:

> What do I enjoy doing?
>
> What do people say I'm good at?
>
> What kinds of activities come naturally to me?
>
> What things make me feel more connected to God and others?
>
> What unique gifts or abilities do I have that others have affirmed in my life?
>
> What experiences from my past equip me with a new perspective?
>
> What ways of serving others make me feel alive?

Take some time to sit down with your journal and reflect. Ask a few close friends to offer their input as well. Try different service opportunities, all the while asking the Holy Spirit to reveal to you in what ways your spiritual gifts can best glorify Him. You may be surprised by what you discover.

Being liberated from a preoccupation with food, we are now free to live justified and satisfied in Christ, embracing the purpose for which God created us with discipline, perseverance, authenticity, and perspective.

Run for the Prize

We admire athletes who break world records. We may even envy them, but if we tried to imitate them without proper training, we would soon encounter resistance. My muscles ache after ten pushups. My lungs burn after two miles. My knees buckle after lifting even half my bodyweight.

Yet each person who achieves greatness pushes through their discomfort to pursue their goal. Their eyes are on their prize, and its brilliance eclipses the momentary pain that screams at them to stop. The apostle Paul says this is similar to Christians' pursuit of their heavenly prize: oneness in Christ.

But this requires daily dedication, and Paul tries to help the church in Corinth understand what that looks like by using athletic imagery that they would have been familiar with:

> Do you not know that in a race all the runners run, but only one gets the prize? Run in such a way as to get the prize. Everyone who competes in the games goes into strict training. They do it to get a crown that will not

last, but we do it to get a crown that will last forever. Therefore I do not run like someone running aimlessly; I do not fight like a boxer beating the air. No, I strike a blow to my body and make it my slave so that after I have preached to others, I myself will not be disqualified for the prize. (1 Corinthians 9:24–27)

Those who hunger and thirst for God will be satisfied with Him, getting both a taste here and now and enjoying the great banquet in heaven. While our salvation is secure in Christ, our heavenly rewards are contingent on our faithfulness here on earth. This is why Paul says the stakes are so high, because we are either completely, absolutely, totally, unequivocally, solely satisfied in Jesus Christ, or we are not satisfied at all. And our satisfaction will inform how we live our lives, how we eat, and what story we tell the world about Christ's redemption.

This all requires discipline. There will be times when you run to food for solace . . . but don't give in to temptation. Run to Jesus instead. We may feel like reading Scripture is too burdensome . . . but don't allow the enemy to lure you into complacency; keep digging into God's Word. You will want to give in to your cravings . . . but don't let them master you. Practice your freedom to say no. We all have times when we hear but choose to tune out the Spirit's warnings . . . but let's not ignore the one who set us free. Listen to Him.

If we want to achieve the prize we're racing for, we must do the hard things, even when that means disciplining our bodies. Jesus told His disciples, "Whoever wants to be my disciple must deny themselves and take up their cross daily and follow me" (Luke 9:23). There's an element of hardship, resistance, and pain

> *God's yes is always better than whatever I said no to before. Whatever I thought I wanted pales in comparison to God's surpassingly beautiful plans.*

there. Paul went so far as to say, "I have been crucified with Christ. It is no longer I who live, but Christ who lives in me" (Galatians 2:20 ESV).

The Christian race is a life of saying no to myself so I can say yes to what God wants for me. And God's yes is always better than whatever I said no to before. Whatever I thought I wanted pales in comparison to God's surpassingly beautiful plans.

So even though my no may feel painful in the moment (especially when the temptation to indulge in that yummy-looking treat seems so overpowering), it paves the way to saying yes to God's better plans and experiencing greater satisfaction in Him. Day, after day, after day.

Digest the Truth
(for individual or group response)

1. How has perfectionism influenced your food fixation?

2. What does Jesus' sacrifice have to do with our struggle to overcome food fixation?

3. What role do self-discipline and grace play in overcoming food fixation?

4. In your journey toward healthy living, have you ever

relapsed into old habits? What did that look like? Has your desire to be perfect for God added shame and guilt to your journey? Do you view relapses as a failure or just a temporary setback? How can relapses actually help you move forward in your pursuit of real comfort in God?

5. Do you believe there is a difference between a "slip" and "relapse" on your journey to food freedom?

Bonus Online Content

Download several beautiful lockscreens to use on your phone or tablet to remind you of The Full Life principles at http://www.thefull.life/lock-screens.

Joanna's story

The first time I became aware of ingredients in food I was around sixteen, standing in the food court at the mall, completely puzzled by the "No MSG" sign above the Chinese food restaurant. That marked the beginning of my food journey, and over the years I've learned more about food, including how it influences our mood, health, and energy.

We're part of a generation that's becoming more aware of our food choices and how they impact our health, but like anything else, healthy living can become an idol in our lives. When we're passionate about something and share that passion with others, we sometimes have a hard time realizing when our passion has become an obsession.

My constant struggle with food in relation to my Christian walk is balance. I try to minister to others—who may not be as far along in their food journey—with graciousness, while at the same time faithfully stewarding this body God has given me to care for as a temple for His Holy Spirit.

I need to constantly remind myself that my life does not ultimately depend on eating or not eating certain foods. Our lives are in God's hands and He has already numbered our days. I need to be sensitive to His guidance in feeding my family and serving others, but my joy and peace about our health and our future cannot come from what I eat or don't eat. My joy and peace are in God.

Part Four

Living
the Full Life

10

Embrace the
Grace of Community

I stared at the screen in disbelief as I read the news report: "Young adults who regularly attend church are 50 percent more likely than their peers to be obese by the time they reach middle age."[1]

Surely I hadn't read that right.

So I read it again. And again. And again. Until the words were seared on my heart.

Tears of grief turned into anger and then hopelessness. How is it possible that the church is contributing to so many of the people wrestling with this problem, especially when we're the ones holding the key to the solution in our pew Bibles?

Rather than being a shining beacon in the darkness of this national epidemic, the church has fallen into a discouraging

FULL: Food, Jesus, and the Battle for Satisfaction

cycle. As the bride of Christ, we can no longer afford to ignore this problem. Let's humbly admit that we're obviously doing something very wrong and we need the Lord to help us, as a faith community, make determined steps toward finding fullness in Christ alone.

The Church-Approved Sin

His eyebrows shot up as he sucked in his belly.

"Food addiction, huh?" he grinned, patting his stomach half in jest. I nodded as the pastor and I shuffled forward in the buffet line. It seemed as though whenever I shared about my writing project, people deflected the seriousness of the topic with self-deprecating humor. It's not that they don't take it seriously. Most people do. They realize the power that food has over them and they wish it would be different. But for some, it's not *that* big of a deal, is it? But it is.

Here's the thing: it doesn't matter if your weakness is Twinkies, organic almonds, coffee, diet soda, alcohol, or any other food substance—if you're controlled by food, you're not controlled by the Holy Spirit.

Ouch.

Does that strike a nerve?

It's uncomfortable, but it's the truth. Paul says it this way: "Do not get drunk on wine, which leads to debauchery. Instead, be filled with the Spirit" (Ephesians 5:18). Interestingly, he juxtaposes drunkenness with being Spirit-filled. Either we're controlled by the Holy Spirit of God or we're controlled by something else. And don't think Paul takes issue with alcohol here exclusively—the point he's making is that if a substance (food or otherwise) leads to debauchery (a fancy word that in the original Greek means *wild extravagance that's careless and foolish*), the Spirit of God does not control that heart. We are slaves to whatever we allow to control us (2 Peter 2:19).

> So I say, walk by the Spirit, and you will not gratify the desires of the flesh. For the flesh desires what is contrary to the Spirit, and the Spirit what is contrary to the flesh. They are in conflict with each other, so that you are not to do whatever you want. (Galatians 5:16–17)

"Oh, but it's not like church potlucks lead to debauchery," I've heard people say. "I mean, alcohol, yes. When you get drunk, you lose control and do things you regret later. But food? Eh, what's the harm?"

Plenty, according to Paul. The word he uses for debauchery in this passage means more than just sexual lewdness; it means "spiritual *wastefulness* due to excessive behavior and the *dire consequences* it brings."[2] If you've ever experienced stomach pain from overeating, if you've ever acted selfishly in eating the last piece of dessert, if you've ever eaten more than you intended to, if you've ever taken your sadness to an ice cream bowl instead of to Jesus, that definition should resonate with you. So although he's using alcohol as a case in point, Paul is speaking here about *any* food or substance that hijacks our command center and causes us to lose control of our actions. You can't be controlled by both food and the Spirit. And for Christians, that statement should jolt some sense into us.

The first time I understood that truth, I was at a baby shower, surrounded by church friends bingeing on select delicacies. This particular church is well-known for its hospitality, and it can throw a party better than any other church I know. In fact, some people attend events here *just* for the food. They wouldn't admit that, of course, but try cutting in front of them in the potluck line and you'll be shot through with an icy glare.

The friend across from me returned to our table with her plate piled high with dessert. She laughed as she sat down. "I only meant to take two, but everything looked so good I had to have one of each," she explained. I nodded empathetically. I know the feeling.

Just then, another friend passed us ready to hit the dessert table for a second round. "The diet begins tomorrow, right, ladies?" she said with a grin. We all laughed. After all, which of us hasn't used that very line to justify our powerlessness before the lure of chocolate eclair, strawberry cheesecake, and other choice foods? *No one here is judging*, the underlying current ran. *We're all in this together.*

Let's not be so quick to run off to heaven that we treat our bodies like disposable paper bags.

And I get that. Really, I do. Food can have such a strong hold over us that it's hard to even recognize the collateral damage in our lives, especially if we hold to platonic dualism—the belief that our spirit is more sacred than our bodies—in an effort to justify unhealthy eating habits. One pastor shared with me a story about a man in his church who had been diabetic for fifteen years but continued to eat whatever he wanted. To offset his poor eating choices, he took more insulin than he was supposed to, and he died an early death because of diabetes. Sadly, many of us in the church continue to eat as if our food choices are of no consequence.

But we are called by God to live on earth with our eyes set on eternity. What would it look like to step toward the full life God offers us while we're still here on earth? How should the fact that we were created in the image of God (with physical bodies) inform the way we steward these vessels? And how can the reality of our future heavenly *glorified yet still physical* bodies affect how we live within these temporal bodies? Let's not be so quick to escape to heaven that we treat our bodies like disposable paper bags, because our physicality has repercussions on our spirituality and vice versa, as we discussed in chapter 1. And that reality is a good thing to keep in mind as we navigate these issues together.

Harnessing the Grace of Community

For all its shortcomings, the church is still God's chosen vessel for spreading the gospel of Christ. And when God makes a plan, you can bet it's a good one. Let's not get disheartened by worrying statistics; instead, let's allow God's Spirit to use the church as the birthplace of healing. Here are some ideas to get started.

Foster Intentional Conversations

I hope this book spurs you on to riveting discussions about ways we can seek fullness in Christ in all areas of our lives: in church halls, in our homes, and in our communities. To that end, I encourage you to seek out opportunities for authentic conversations on this topic. What might this look like within the church community, practically speaking?

Talk with your pastor and get his perspective on the issue. Read widely from different Christian traditions to learn what others have to say. Seek out people in your faith community who are eager to study and engage with Scripture on a variety of topics, including food issues.

And use social media for good. Rather than engage in drivel, redeem the social space for conversations that make people pause, ponder, and posit. In the writing of this book, I often wrestled with questions I wasn't quite sure how to answer, and rather than go with my first instinct, I reached out to my Facebook friends to get their thoughts. Those threads contributed rich conversations, and my heart smiled to see my friends from around the world (most of whom didn't know each other) engage in friendly conversations, pointing out fallacies in each other's thinking, and building on one another's thoughts. It was an incredibly rewarding experience and contributed several of the finer points shared in this book.

We need to be having these conversations in safe places, free from judgment and prejudice. Let's not assume that everyone who is overweight struggles with food issues; it is not our duty to read spiritual issues into physical conditions. It is the Holy Spirit's job to convict, and it's our job to love and walk together in obedience and recovery.

Study Scripture to Form a Biblical Theology of Food

For too long we've allowed the secular world to tell us what we should believe about food. And while we can learn much from science about the intricate ways God created our bodies, the medical community can offer only a limited perspective of how God created us to use and enjoy food.

What we believe about food informs our view of God. And the converse is also true: what we believe about God informs our view of food. So let's begin to develop a food theology, a study of God and food so that we can grow in our love and worship of God and learn to appreciate food as the gift God meant it to be.

Begin studying Scripture for yourself, asking God to help you see and understand His plan for food in your life. Use a concordance to look up verses about food, eating, gluttony, satisfaction, fullness, and similar keywords. As you read stories in the Bible, notice what role food played in their interactions and what you can learn from each of their stories (think of Adam and Eve, Esau and Jacob, Joseph and the Egyptians, Ruth and Boaz, Abigail and David, Jonathan and the honeycomb, the widow and Elijah). As you immerse yourself in the Word of God, He will begin transforming your view of food, and your understanding and love for God will change as well.

And then share what you're learning with your faith community. Allow these stories to enter your conversations in the church hallways while discussing recipes and diets. If the Word of God is living and active (Hebrews 4:12), then we can trust it to shape our churches as we welcome it in our midst.

Feed the Hungry

What if the solution to the American church obesity problem is also the solution to the global hunger epidemic?

It sounds crazy to think that we could solve world hunger, but think of this: there are 318.86 million people in the United States,[3] of which 39 percent report being highly active in their faith community, attending church every week.[4] As we've already established, the American church, overall, has an overeating problem. We simply eat too much. (On the whole, we eat a lot of junk food too, but when it comes down to it, we have an obesity problem because *we eat too much food.*) On average, US households spend $550.00 a month on groceries and eating out.[5] (That number varies widely based on a number of factors, but feel free to calculate your own monthly food budget and follow along.)

What would happen if we fasted from a meal once a week and prayerfully gave that money to world organizations that feed the hungry? I'll tell you what would happen: hungry people would be fed and fed-up people would hunger for righteousness. It's as simple as that. In fact, donating the cost of one steak dinner can feed five children for a month. A month! If just 20 percent of American church attenders ate less and gave more, we could go a long way toward solving world hunger.[6]

Every time we curb our appetites to feed those in need, we're essentially feeding Jesus.

Now I know that many of you reading this book give faithfully, regularly, and generously to a number of charitable causes already, so I'm not trying to guilt anyone into donating more money to charity. But here is what I *am* saying: God has entrusted us with the resources needed to solve global hunger—and we're selfishly squandering them on our own unquenchable appetites. While precious people around the world go hungry, we're complaining when our jeans fit too tightly.

Recall the story Jesus told of the rich man who had a plentiful harvest and built larger barns to store more stuff so he could "take life easy" and "eat, drink, and be merry." Remember how that story ends? The man dies that very night and Jesus calls him and everyone else like him "fools" because they "store up things for themselves but [are] not rich toward God" (Luke 12:13–21). And one of the ways we can be rich toward God, storing up treasures in heaven instead of packing on the pounds here on earth, is by recognizing the opportunity to serve Jesus by serving others: "I was hungry and you gave me something to eat, I was thirsty and you gave me something to drink" (Matthew 25:35). Every time we curb our appetites to feed those in need, we're essentially feeding Jesus.

The church my family attends does a beautiful job of fleshing this out in a very practical way. The Chapel in Green, Ohio, partners with local ministries in Yucatan, Mexico, to equip leaders, establish churches, and extend mercies. One of the practical ways we serve them is by packing nutritional rice bags to provide meals to the Mayan people. For several years now, our church leaders have distributed yellow paper buses to church attendees and encouraged us to keep the bus on our kitchen table, praying for the ministry every day and placing a dollar in the box every evening. At the end of the challenge, we bring our buses back to the church, filled with donations and covered in prayer, and together we pack meals that will feed hungry families in Mexico.

Perhaps one of the easiest ways to turn our food fixation outside in is to stop worrying about losing weight and focus instead on feeding those who desperately need to put on weight. Even if your church doesn't organize a similar feed-the-hungry campaign, create your own. Commit to spending 5 or 10 percent less on groceries this month, and donate the amount you saved to an organization that will feed hungry children. Or skip one morning latte a week and give that savings to your local shelter's meal ministry. Or get the family involved and use that money to make peanut butter and jelly sandwiches you can distribute to the homeless in your downtown area. And do it again next month. And the month after that. And so on.

Whatever you do, make a habit of feeding the hungry from your own plate, and over time you may discover that you yourself eat less so that those who have none may have more. And in the process, we will learn that indeed, it is better to give than to receive (Acts 20:35).

Offer Healthy Choices

As I was discussing this chapter with my husband, he remarked on the donuts that grace the worship team's side table every Sunday morning. As part of the worship band, he and others get to church at 7:30 a.m. to prepare for that day's set. And God bless those sweet souls who provide morning treats for the crew!

It's a thoughtful gesture, and one everyone appreciates all around. But as we were discussing the obesity epidemic inside the church, Flaviu remarked that those who typically bring food to church gatherings—whether post-sermon coffee-and-pastry time, potluck dinners, church picnics, pancake breakfast fundraisers, or Sunday sundae socials—have the power to change the food culture in our churches.

Pastor Dave Fisher describes what this change looked like in his church: "We started putting out healthy food. Fruits, apples, granola bars, and water for early morning meetings so people could eat healthier in the morning. We did the same thing with our kids, offering healthy snacks in the classrooms instead of candy and chocolates. At first people asked, 'Where's the donuts?' and we said, 'We're trying to help people eat healthier, so we don't serve those.' And surprisingly, the congregation reacted really well."[7]

Some of the creative programs churches can offer include food addiction recovery support groups, healthy cooking classes, exercise classes, and Bible studies on food.

In other words, we need to be the change we want to see. There's no way I'm going to ask those darling souls to stop bringing donuts to the band room on Sunday mornings. What they're doing is heartfelt and sincere and, let's be honest, there are days that simply call for enjoying friends' company with the food set before us. But perhaps, in my tiny corner of influence, when I get asked to bring something to a small group gathering, I'll forgo my standby brownies and bring a fruit salad instead.

Look for opportunities to make small changes that will move your local church and the surrounding community in the right direction over time. These will be unique to your community and your church. Some of the creative programs churches can offer include food addiction recovery support groups, healthy cooking classes, exercise classes, and Bible studies on food. These are great ideas, but be aware that what works for one church may not work for another. Earnestly seek the Spirit's direction to see what He wants to do in your community. Then do it. You may be surprised at the doors that open before you.

As Pastor Steve Willis began addressing food addiction in his church and leading initiatives to help his congregation care for their bodies as the temples of God, he saw more and more opportunities to be a testimony locally in their community and even nationally: "The greatest thing to me throughout this whole process is God has taken something that even our fallen culture understands is a problem. The world knows this is an issue, and they want the church to speak out on these issues of justice. I have been able to share the good news about Christ and how the Bible is relevant today to hundreds of people who would never step into a church."[8]

What if this can become a unique opportunity for the Holy Spirit to move powerfully in and through us?

Many people have long been praying for a revival in the church; perhaps that revival will begin with a surrender on this very issue. God desires to stir in us such a hunger and thirst for Him that we will turn from the temptations our enemy dangles before us and feast on God's Word. Imagine the changes that would take place one life at a time in our congregations, our communities, and our world if we surrender our appetites and seek satisfaction in God alone.

He can do it. He is able.

Digest the Truth
(*for individual or group response*)

1. How can the church come alongside individuals struggling with food issues while still remaining committed to biblical evangelism and discipleship?

2. What are some creative ways ministry leaders can use to encourage a holistic view of discipleship (body, soul, and spirit)? Or is discipleship exclusively concerned with training the spirit in holiness (to the exclusion of body and soul)?

3. When Christians struggle with having a proper perspective about food, how might this struggle influence their thinking about God? And conversely, how can an inaccurate view of God influence their thinking about food? How should food passages in the Bible influence how we think and relate to food?

4. Do our food struggles influence our witness to the onlooking unbelieving world? If so, in what way, and how can we better testify to the satisfaction found in Jesus? If not, why not?

5. What practices does the Western church have that create a harmful relationship with food? How can your local church use abundance to serve those who are hungry?

Bonus Online Content

Access more statistics on food and the church, and download a printable to share with your church leaders at http://www.thefull.life/statistics.

Pastor Dave's story

We all have parts of our lives that we tend to ignore and think we'll be okay. Food is one of them.

When I became sober in my twenties, food took the place of alcohol in my life, consuming my thoughts and luring me with its promise of satisfaction. I wasn't concerned about my food addiction because I didn't see the immediate effects of my choices, even as a pastor. It seems we don't take food addiction seriously until a doctor says, "You're going to die if you don't lose weight."

Last year my mentor lost a lot of weight, making me reconsider my own life choices. I was eating for comfort rather than nutrition, and it was affecting my witness to the world. I began to realize that when I'd sit across from a drug addict or alcoholic with a bloated stomach from my last indulgence, I didn't have a place to speak into their lives. Our ministries are built around relationships; to minister authentically, we must be willing to face our own struggles.

In the past six months, I've lost over fifty pounds. But even better, I've gained a greater appetite for God. Our church has implemented several healthy initiatives, and we're seeing a great response among our congregation. As we move forward, we're reaching into our community with the message of hope and satisfaction in Christ, living as healthy followers of Jesus who are completely captivated by Him.

11

Serve with Food

For many people, preparing and serving food is an expression of love. When a girlfriend goes through a hard breakup, we might bring over warm chocolate chip cookies and cry together on the couch. When a child is feeling ill, we might make homemade chicken soup and coax him to health. When a coworker retires after years of service, we might gather around a table laden with food to celebrate her new season in life.

And even if we're not the ones preparing the meal, food somehow still finds its way to the center of our gatherings, whether it's a dinner-and-movie date, a casual get-together for coffee and a chat, or a celebratory outing with the softball team after a tough win. Food seems to be magnetic in its ability to bring people together, for better or for worse.

For many Christians, the term *fellowship* conjures up images of people chatting over coffee and donuts. When it comes to food and fellowship, Christians lead the way. Or so it seems. Too often, food becomes the focal point of our gatherings and fellowship becomes an afterthought, a spiritual label we can slap on our meetings to make them sound more righteous than they are.

Perhaps the best place to start is to define our terms, looking at what it means to fellowship in the first place, and then examining ways food can both foster and hinder fellowship.

Redefining *Fellowship* in Christian Circles

Something magical happens when people gather around a table. Plates are passed. Glasses are refilled. Time stands still. Hearts connect.

One of my favorite pastimes is hosting people in my home. I'll admit I'm not the best cook you'll ever meet (that title goes to my mom, hands down), but I enjoy having my home full of friends as we laugh, reminisce, and dig into steaming bowls of yummy food.

Fellowshipping over food is scriptural. After all, Jesus invited His disciples to fellowship over a breakfast of grilled fish. Just imagine: the Son of God (who spoke the world into existence and created every kind of fish, who crafted the trees to cut down for wood, and invented even the fiery spark of flame itself) prepared a meal of fish, grilled to perfection, for His exhausted disciples who were on a fishing expedition. I imagine that was the best-tasting fish Peter and his cohorts had ever eaten. We know it was a delicious meal, not only because everything Jesus did was perfect, but also because the water Jesus turned into wine at a wedding was better than the best wine in the region.

Jesus often was found lingering over a meal with old and

new friends. In fact, when the Pharisees were looking for dirt on Him, they accused Him of being a "glutton and a drunkard" (Matthew 11:19), which we know is not true because in all His eating and drinking, Jesus never sinned. But He did enjoy meals in people's houses, and as a traveling prophet, He would have had many occasions to eat both simple meals on the road and elaborate meals in the homes of the rich.

How can we prioritize biblical fellowship in our interactions with one another, especially when gathered around the table?

As we discussed in the previous chapter, twenty-first-century churches have readily adopted this practice of gathering around meals. But in a society obsessed with food and riddled with food issues, we may have allowed our preoccupation with food to replace fellowship as the focal point of our get-togethers. Due to the prevalence of food addictions, obsessions, and sensitivities in our culture, Christians today must learn new ways to connect, fellowship, and minister to others in ways that are creative, personal, and intentional, whether they involve food or not.

In Acts 2:42, we're told that the first-century church devoted themselves not only to the apostles' teaching and prayer, but also to fellowship and the breaking of bread.

The term used in Scripture for fellowship is *koinonia*, a Greek word meaning "fellowship, association, community, communion, joint participation, intercourse."[1]And while food is often present in these gatherings, it's not just about eating but about sharing with each other blessings and burdens, privileges, responsibilities, common goals, and visions.

In the Bible, fellowship goes in two directions: vertical—communion with the Lord through Scripture, prayer, and walking in the Spirit; and horizontal—communion with believers. We get together with fellow Christians, worshiping together and sharing needs, burdens, concerns, joys, and blessings. We encourage one another as well as comfort, challenge, exhort, pray with and for each other, and provide practical help according to needs and ability (see Philippians 1:27, 2:4; Romans 12:15; 1 Thessalonians 5:11–15).

The goal is to enrich one another with the things of Christ as we do life together, sharing with each other the good and the bad as we become more like Christ.

In Romans 12, Paul gives us a picture of what this kind of fellowship looks like fleshed out in community daily life:

Love must be sincere. Hate what is evil; cling to what is good. Be devoted to one another in love. Honor one another above yourselves. Never be lacking in zeal, but keep your spiritual fervor, serving the Lord. Be joyful in hope, patient in affliction, faithful in prayer. Share with the Lord's people who are in need. Practice hospitality. Bless those who persecute you; bless and do not curse. Rejoice with those who rejoice; mourn with those who mourn. Live in harmony with one another. Do not be proud, but be willing to associate with people of low position. Do not be conceited. (vv. 9–16)

The entire chapter speaks of community life in fellowship, and we could take an entire chapter to unpack just these eight verses. But the overarching question that concerns us is this: How can we prioritize biblical fellowship in our interactions with one another, especially when gathered around the table?

From the text directly, here are a few practical ways we can apply Paul's teaching in the context of food:

Love each other with food in ways that proceed from genuine feelings. In other words, check your motives before bringing that fancy appetizer to the weekend party. Make sure you're not just looking for compliments. If you're going to love with food, then make sure you're actually loving and not just using food as a pretense to show off your culinary skills.

Engage trending food stories critically. When reading an article about food (whether it's a new recipe or a fad diet or an exposé on the dangers of sugar), think carefully about the messages communicated. Are there any subtle lies trying to infiltrate your thinking? Is the author using fearmongering to co-opt you into a specific action (like buying their product)? Throw out what's evil and cling to what's good.

When serving a meal, focus on the people in front of you. What are they going through? What burdens are they shouldering? What good news are they celebrating? Remember that even a cold cup of water given in Jesus' name is received by Him. Serve the meal as unto the Lord, and look for ways for your guests to feel seen, known, and loved.

Let meals become about more than just filling stomachs with food. Make the table a safe place where each person can share in each other's joys and pains. Foster conversations that go beyond surface pleasantries and allow for deeper soul-knowing to take place.

Seek to understand rather than be understood. When interacting with those who have experienced food addiction or food disorders, or who may have particular food allergies or sensitivities, be patient and loving. Invite them to share as much as they are comfortable.

Be faithful in praying for each other in the areas of food addiction, food fixation, food disorders, and food shortage.

Look for opportunities to steward your surplus to serve those facing a need. All around the world and down the street, people are going hungry. Perhaps there are ways to reduce your food budget so that others may go to bed with full bellies.

Open your home with generosity and friendliness. Practice receiving and entertaining guests, visitors, and strangers with welcoming arms. And don't worry about what's for dinner; whether it's a five-course meal or a five-dollar pizza, remember that the point is not the food but the people. Don't allow food to stress you; as long as it won't make people sick, it will all be good.

Refuse to get drawn into food fights. Not the rotten-apple kind but the rotten-word kind, the ones where social media channels become virtual cafeterias for people to fling hurtful insults to those whose food philosophies differ from their own. Act kindly toward those who have diametrically opposite views; vegans can indeed be friends with meat-lovers.

Be mindful of others' food sensitivities to ensure you use food to bless those around you instead of causing them harm. It doesn't take much effort to ask if there are any food allergies you should be aware of, and your gluten-free guests will thank you for your thoughtfulness.

Serve others with food. Food finds its way into both celebration and mourning, and for good reason: a shared meal crosses language, cultural, and emotional barriers. Take a pot of soup to the mom who's just had a baby and to the one who's lost her baby. Sit next to the one who's hurting; make her tea just the way she likes it and let the tears slip in silence. Celebrate the big and small accomplishments in life, because a shared ice cream cone over making the volleyball team or finishing a master's class makes others feel seen and known.

Live in harmony with those who have different food philosophies from you. Don't just tolerate them, but recognize how different elements can come together in beautiful combinations. Learn about food traditions around the world. Try new recipes from other countries. Introduce your kids to a typical meal in the country your sponsored child lives in. Don't make a fuss if you can't eat the main dish your hostess serves because she forgot you're a vegetarian.

Invite people into your home and at your table, especially those who are overlooked by others (see Luke 14:12–13). Reach out to international students at your local university who can't go home for the holidays. Drive over to pick up the shut-in who hasn't shared a meal with anyone but the TV in weeks. Become friends with the veteran sitting on the street corner and fill his belly with warm food. Open your home and open your heart.

Be humble, modest, and respectful of others' needs, views, and opinions of food. Entertain the notion that you might have something to learn from the unlikeliest of people, and actively seek opportunities to interact with those who are different from you.

As you can see, this passage alone from Romans 12 could radically transform our views on and interactions with food. Food, though one of the most basic common denominators among people (because everyone needs to eat to survive), can be one of the greatest differentiators (because everyone has so many different preferences, beliefs, and practices).

What can we learn from this passage about prioritizing fellowship in our eating together, sharing recipes, talking about the latest fad diets, and learning from one another about cultural food differences? How can we serve with food, allowing this good gift from God to become a vehicle of edification both inside the church and out into the world? How could an intentional food theology and philosophy affect the way we serve one another? How could we incorporate this idea of fellowship over food to promote the gospel and build up believers?

One church I knew of was very intentional in its use of food in this way. Every Saturday evening, members of the small church gathered together around slow cookers and casserole dishes, not just to fellowship with one another but also to invite the community into their midst. They reached out to neighbors, homeless veterans, placeless college students, and anyone who was looking for friendly company. They would always make more food than they needed and invited more people than they thought they could feed, but somehow the food was always enough, and having filled their stomachs, they created space in the conversation to nourish their souls as well.

This church, made up of ragamuffins and philosophy professors, bohemian students and the upper crust class represented a beautiful portrait of heaven: a place where people from every strata of society, every walk of life, and every nation of the world will gather together around tables laden with food to celebrate the marriage of Jesus to His bride. What a party! What delight for both stomach and soul! What nourishment— both of temporal delicacies and eternal delights.

Are you surprised that food is featured in the description of what we have to look forward to in heaven? Have you ever thought of what it will be like to sit down to dinner with Ruth, Bathsheba, Rahab, and others in the genealogy of Jesus? And not just for a metaphorical meal but for the best delicacies the universe has ever seen, all while enjoying fellowship with God and each other, unhindered by pride, worry, distractions, or second thoughts. This beautiful scene is what we preview when we share in the communion meal, and to a lesser degree, when we commune over a meal.

Serving One Another with Food

It's said that the way to a man's heart is through his stomach, and for many marriages that might be true. In my marriage, however, it's the other way around. Whereas I tend toward food fixation, my husband, Flaviu, would more aptly be described as having a food indifference. He couldn't care less whether his dinner is filet mignon or boxed mac and cheese—it's all food to him.

I, however, have developed a taste for the finer things in life, and an ideal date would be a nice sit-down meal at a restaurant we haven't been to before, followed by a detailed conversation regarding the ingredients featured in each course and the cooking methods employed to reach the perfect finish on each dish. Needless to say, our different views of food have been the cause of many a marital conversation, especially around special events and anniversaries, and while early in our marriage this used to frustrate me to no end, I have come to appreciate my husband's different view of food.

> The heart of hospitality is about creating space for someone to feel seen and heard and loved. It's about declaring your table a safe zone, a place of warmth and nourishment. Part of that, then, is honoring the way God made our bodies, and feeding them in the ways they need to be fed.[2]

There are ways to serve and love with food and without food. Obviously, making sure there's food in the house for three meals a day is one way to serve my husband with food (though he would gladly grab dinner straight out of the fridge and eat it standing at the kitchen counter without even heating it). Getting special foods to mark special events is another. Like the time we celebrated our anniversary by getting an international cheese platter, complete with five hard-to-pronounce cheeses, jams, and crackers, and driving to a local park for a low-key picnic. Or the time we saved up several months' worth of date money to go to a prestigious steakhouse where we looked at the menus and chuckled over the outrageous prices (but it's still the best steak I've had to this day).

We practice that hospitality first and foremost in our families, using food as a vehicle to deepen relationships with our spouses and children. Here are some ideas:

Plan healthy meals that nourish your family.

Prioritize family dinners. If your family is always grabbing food on the go, start with one family dinner night, and add in more as is feasible. Keep the fare simple, but make the conversations intentional. Ask everyone to share.

Invite your kids into the kitchen and cook together. They will not only learn the basics of making a nutritious meal but you'll also make fond memories that they'll cherish over the years.

Look for reasons to celebrate together around the table. Make a toast. Pop the sparkling grape juice. Set the table with the fine china. Fold the napkins into fancy designs.

We can also practice hospitality by inviting people into our homes and making space for them at our tables. It's not so much about entertaining guests as it is about enveloping them with warmth and a welcoming attitude. Although setting out the fine china and special floral arrangements is definitely touching, there's something to be said about "scruffy hospitality" as well. People come over to see and spend time with you for who you are, so don't worry so much about a three-course dinner. Focus your attention instead on those precious ones walking across your doorstep. How can you help carry their burdens? How can you make them feel seen and heard and just a tad less burdened because they spent time with you?

Food naturally binds people together, and it's a great way to create shared memories.

Food-Free Friendship and Fellowship

Just a few days after our second daughter was born, we realized she had a rare form of jaundice that wasn't responding to typical treatment. I was in the NICU, helplessly standing by as our little one was strapped up to machines and surrounded by three ultraviolet therapy units (because the two they started her on were not lowering her bilirubin fast enough).

In the midst of the flurry of activity, I posted a picture to Facebook and asked friends to pray. Minutes later a friend from church texted me and offered to come to the hospital to stay with me. She even offered to bring me a Starbucks drink (sugar-free, because we were both participating in a forty-day sugar fast). In that moment, even just *knowing* that someone would come stand with me was comforting, and her presence was the best gift I could have asked for.

But when it's my turn to offer comfort to friends, I've got to admit my mind first flies to comfort food. And that's sometimes an entirely appropriate response. But there are other times that call for creative ways of showing love that don't center around food, like when your best friend goes through a break-up but is sticking to her low-carb diet. (Chocolate chip cookies? Nope. Chocolate-covered pretzels? No way. Bananas? Lame.)

These are great opportunities to step back and reassess what it means to offer comfort, how you can alleviate grief or pain in ways that mean the most to that person. Think through the 5 *Love Languages*[3] and brainstorm ways you can love in those situations. Here are just a few ideas: Write a heartfelt note expressing what you cherish about your friendship. Pick up a potted plant from the store. Frame a picture of the two of you having fun. Offer to go for a walk together, either to talk or not.

As we learn to become creative, intentional, and personal in fostering fellowship, we will find it gets easier. And with time, we may be the ones introducing others to food-free fellowship ideas.

I'll never forget the shock I felt the first time I attended a Bible study in someone's house and there was nothing to eat. Nothing. I had come hungry because I was expecting a spread (because that's how we Romanians do it). But all my new friend offered us was water and tea. Don't get me wrong—the tea was fabulous and the water was refreshing, but where were the finger foods? Nowhere in sight.

Over the weeks that followed, I learned that this sweet woman omitted food intentionally because she found that food often got in the way of fellowship. By the end of the study, I was relieved there was no food, because there were no food thoughts to distract me. *I don't want to be the first one to take a piece. Oh good. She took one and so did she, so now I can help myself. Did everyone only take one? Would it be rude to take two? Maybe I should wait a few minutes. Okay, can I go for seconds now?* What a gift to be able to walk into the room and look around at the faces of the women gathered instead of immediately checking what's to eat. It's a lesson I won't soon forget.

When Your Loved One has a Food Addiction

One of the hardest places to be is on the outside of a food addiction looking in. As I've been writing this book, several women have confided in me the struggle they're facing trying to help their spouse or child who struggles with food fixation.

This common theme seemed to follow me wherever I went. In fact, one time I was being wheeled out of the hospital after a minor procedure. When the orderly found out the topic of my book, she broke down in tears, sharing her story right there in front of the hospital double doors as we awaited my ride. This petite twenty-something told me about her ex-husband, who had lost one hundred pounds and had become so consumed with his eating and exercise routines that everything else in his life faded away. "I fell to about number five on his priorities list, and he simply didn't have time or interest for anything other than his weight-loss program," she said. This neglect made her feel like she was a burden rather than a partner, and contributed to her decision to seek a divorce after a few short years of marriage.

It doesn't matter if the obsession is around eating food or not eating food. Food fixation, in any form, can become such a preoccupation that it consumes one's entire attention, affection, energy, and devotion, leaving other relationships suffering in its wake.

If you're in this situation, you know what a lonely and hopeless place it can be as you watch your loved one battle this stronghold. First and foremost, make sure they know Christ as their personal Savior; they will never find fullness and satisfaction outside of Him.

Here are some other practical steps you can take to help:

Pray Unceasingly

As much as you'd like to jump in right away and make drastic changes, pause and pray. One of the greatest problems of food fixation is denying there's a problem in the first place. Resist the temptation to nag or point out all the ways they're "doing it wrong." Chances are you've tried this in the past and failed, and that's because only the Spirit of God can convict of sin.

Ask God to give you wisdom and patience as you begin this journey toward fullness in Christ with your loved one. It may be long and trying but it's also rewarding. And you'll need God to help you stay the course.

Seek to Understand

For someone who doesn't struggle with food fixation, it can be really hard to understand why the offending person can't just "shape up." It can be frustrating when they try a new diet program with great hopes, only to fail. Reserve judgment and seek first to understand them. What are the circumstances surrounding their upbringing that may predispose them to certain food-abusive behaviors? What triggers a binge? What lies are they believing that they need to overcome with truth?

This is a treasure hunt not a witch hunt. The more you understand about your loved one, the better able you'll be to help them along the way.

Get Help

If they're willing, connect them with the help they need to succeed. This might be counseling, a support group, or resources. Educate yourselves about how food fuels the body and how food addiction short-circuits normal brain functions. Learn how to cook healthy meals and spend time together creating fun and memorable dishes.

As a side note, *you* also need a support group, whether

that's a trusted friend you can call when you've reached your wits' end or another woman who is walking this road to recovery alongside her own loved one.

Walk Alongside

While God frees some people immediately, most of us experience a gradual freeing as we walk in obedience to God and seek Him. Come alongside your loved one and walk the path of food freedom with them. Celebrate the wins together and be willing to adapt as new seasons bring new challenges.

Above All, Love Regardless

Food fixation is often rooted in deep insecurities and fears that surface in myriad ways, some of them more painful than others. Reassure them that you love them and will stand by them no matter what.

Because of issues I had witnessed in some people's marriages, I carried with me a fear that Flaviu would leave me if I gained weight. When I was pregnant with Carissa, I was terrified as I watched the pounds pile on late in my pregnancy, but Flaviu tenderly and graciously reassured me of his steadfast love and relentless commitment to my and our baby's health. With both pregnancies, he helped me stay active by taking me out for evening walks and cutting up apples so I had healthy snacks on hand. He listened to me as I complained about the stretch marks and told me how beautiful he thought my body was when carrying his children.

And he stayed close to my side as I stumbled my way toward finding abundant joy and satisfaction in God.

Digest the Truth

(*for individual or group response*)

1. How can you structure life activities (family celebrations, date nights, church activities) in ways that focus on people and not food?

2. How does food show up in the afterlife? In what ways will we eat and drink in the new heaven and new earth?

3. What are some ideas in the chapter you can try? What have you seen others do?

4. Has someone ever served you with food? What was your reaction?

Bonus Online Content

Watch Asheritah share practical ways to serve with food, and download "7 Tips to Help a Loved One Struggling with Food Fixation" at http://www.thefull.life/help-loved-one.

Ana's story

After my second daughter was born, I knew I had to change something: I wasn't feeling well, I was struggling to lose the baby weight, and I just had no energy.

I had heard that food influences our health, so I started researching what goes into the food I eat and how to eat in a healthy manner. That process took months, and I gradually adjusted the way I ate and fed my family.

But change wasn't always easy. I specifically remember two or three instances when I absolutely crashed. I had set goals many times before and wasn't able to reach them, but I wanted this time to be different. So I said, "Lord, I can't do this by myself. You're going to have to help me." And He did. God gave me strength and helped me remove what was unhealthy, restore what was possible, and rebuild my life.

I learned to make healthy choices, one meal at a time. And when I made mistakes, I didn't allow disappointment and guilt to drag me down. This time around, I got back up and kept moving.

There was a point though when I realized I was becoming consumed by healthy eating, because most of my thoughts and time were spent trying to make the healthiest choice possible for our family. I was reminded of Jesus' words that `life is more than food` (Luke 12:23) and healthy eating. So again I prayed, asking the Holy Spirit to fill me with His fire and give me His desires. And again He answered. He empowered me to stick to healthy routines while shifting my thoughts, energy, and attention toward Him, and every day He fills me with joy as I know Him more.

12

Navigate Seasons of Change

When this book was still a dream in my heart, I found out I was pregnant with my second child.

I was thrilled, of course, but when morning sickness gave way to intense cravings, I began to question my ability to write a book on overcoming food fixation. I thought I had made such progress after Jesus had set me free from my sugar addiction the year before, so how come I was once again standing at my kitchen counter with the cookie dough ice cream carton in one hand and a spoon in the other? Why was it so hard to overcome the cravings I thought I had defeated and buried in the past? I crawled under the covers in shame and later called my agent to tell her that maybe this was a bad idea.

I took deep breaths and willed myself to speak. I was afraid to even voice my confession, convinced that as soon as she heard about my struggles she would call off the project and revoke our contract. After all, who was I to write a book about overcoming food addiction when I was craving chicken lo mien every night? Shame can do that to us, you know. Keep us quiet and alone, convinced that if the truth comes out, the people closest to us will stop loving us and confirm our worst fears: that we're doomed to a life of failure and that we're naive to dream big dreams.

I held my breath, expecting the worst. But in her kindness, my agent said what I desperately needed to hear but was afraid to believe: "These pregnancy cravings? They don't negate what God has done in you in the past. And they certainly don't disqualify you from writing this book." She continued. "In fact, this is the very reason you need to write this book—not because you've arrived but because you understand the struggle. This struggle *in this very season* is a gift because it forces you to rely on Jesus every day, and that's exactly where you need to be."

This struggle in this season is a gift.

Those words settled deep in my heart, and they breathed hope into my life that these food triggers that threatened to defeat me could actually lead to a season of deeper transformation and sweeter communion with my Savior.

Challenging Seasons of Life

In talking with other women who have walked through seasons of life, I've found that we're often unprepared to face food struggles that slip in through the back door when we're least expecting them. What can we do when the seasons in our lives threaten to undo the progress and growth we've experienced in our walk with God, especially as it pertains to food?

First off, let's look at some of the transitions that commonly trigger an unhealthy food obsession, and why each of them can be so challenging.

College or Independence

After a childhood spent under the vigilant eyes of caring parents, young adults are finally free to make their own choices. And those choices often result in unwanted weight gain. Suddenly, the cafeteria offers myriad and unlimited options, there's no one to tell them to eat their veggies, and dorm life brings with it late-night snacking and pizza deliveries. Freshman Fifteen, here we come!

For others, the pressure to perform both athletically and academically exacerbates eating disorders, and food becomes something the student can control in a world that often seems out-of-control.

Pregnancy

For some women, raging hormones cause the most bizarre cravings, and well-meaning people encourage you to eat whatever you want. (I was even told that if I resisted my cravings, my child could be born with birth defects. Well then, don't mind me if I just eat that whole platter of cookies! I'm acting in the best interest of my child, after all.)

But at the other end of the food obsession spectrum, there's the medical staff who carefully charts our weight gain, the paranoia about eating something that could harm our baby, and the media pressure to get our pre-baby body back in record time. As if that's not enough, your own body is conspiring against you in the months following the birth, holding on to baby weight to secure solid milk production.

Injury or Illness

There you are, happily training for a triathlon when a knee injury forces you onto the sidelines. Okay, more realistically, you probably weren't in the running for the national Olympics team, but even for average women, an injury or debilitating sickness can make us feel like we're on the bench watching the world pass us by. We pack on pounds, not only because we can't engage in our normal physical activities, but because medication often comes with unpleasant side effects like weight gain. Plus, what's more comforting at the end of a hard day than kicking back with a bowl of chips and a good period drama? I've been there and chances are if you haven't yet, you will be at some point in your life.

Life Transitions (marriage, kids, divorce, empty nest, etc.)

Just when you thought you had a handle on a good exercise routine and a healthy food rotation, along comes a major life change that throws everything into chaos. It doesn't matter so much what that transition is as much as how it affects you. Your normal schedule is derailed, and you find yourself grabbing whatever is easily accessible be it fast food, pizza delivery, or a candy bar in the grocery checkout lane. Choosing good food falls way down the list of priorities, and survival mode takes over. It's during times of crisis like this that "just this once" becomes a series of choices leading to bad habits that carry over long after the dust has settled and you find yourself in a new normal.

Holidays

The deadly trifecta (Halloween-Thanksgiving-Christmas) strikes every year, so you'd think we'd have come up with a better way to handle these disturbances to our normal healthy routine. *But there's food everywhere!* And not salads and fruit cups. Holiday parties, family get-togethers, school activities, and clearance shelves beckon that we indulge *just this once* in our seasonal favorites; you can hardly go a day without encountering some food-centered event that's sure to feature seasonal foods, beverages, and flavors you've just *got* to try.

But on the other side of the spectrum, we can be so scared of gaining weight during this time that we become hyper vigilant about our eating, obsessing over what healthy options will be available at these gatherings and slipping into old habits of obsessing over every single bite. And it's not like you can just grit your teeth and get through the end of the year; many New Year resolutions have been derailed by Valentine's Day chocolates, Shamrock Shakes, and Easter candy, leading to a half-hearted "I'll do better next year."

If you've identified one or more of these seasons as past triggers in your own life, take a few moments to reflect on how they affected you then, so that you'll be better prepared to address the triggers in your life now.

Evaluate Your Current Situation

Some transitions in life are very clear, like moving away to college, but others are subtle, like one gloomy day slipping into another before you recognize depression wrapping its cloak around you.

Regardless of whether or not you've anticipated this season in your life, spend some time with the Lord in prayer and ask Him to show you where you're currently struggling. Consider journaling about the events in your life that constantly cause you to trip up.

> What major events or trials are going on in your life right now?
>
> Which specific situations trigger your food fixation? Describe the circumstances and the factors that tempt you to overstep your boundaries (overeating, caloric restriction, obsessively thinking about food, etc.).
>
> What lies about food, God, or yourself are you believing? Have you tried renewing your mind with God's truth? If not, what's keeping you from proactively fighting these lies?
>
> What emotions are you predominantly feeling, especially before acting out your food fixation? How intense are those feelings? How else could you handle those emotions in a way that is safe and healthy?
>
> Have you been spending regular time with God in prayer, the Word, and worship? If not, what specific challenges are you facing that keep you from making this a consistent habit?
>
> Who knows about your current struggles? Have you confessed your failings to God and

a trusted friend? Who could come alongside
you to encourage you in finding fullness in
Christ?

What would your life look like in two or three
months if you continue to eat the way you are
right now? Describe, in detail, where the path
you're walking is taking you. Is that a destination you'd like to reach? If not, what do you
need to do to turn around?

What would your life look like if, instead of
seeking satisfaction in food, you ran to God
with your needs? Which of the specific tools
in this book can you use to help you fight
food fixation and eat from a place of fullness
in Christ?[1]

This journaling exercise will take some time, but it's so
helpful in identifying the unique challenges of the season we're
currently in. After all, we can't come up with creative solutions
if we don't know what the problem is in the first place. Part of
our struggle to transition between seasons is applying solutions that have worked in the past without reassessing the challenges that are unique to a new season.

Reflect on Past Triggers

Next, take each of those triggers described above and think
about previous experiences you've had. Ask the Spirit to help
you see the spiritual struggle behind those situations.

If you can, identify a specific experience that's similar to your current situation and return to that scene in your mind. It's easy to bury those memories in the recesses of our minds, especially when they're heavy with guilt and regret. But rather than ignore them and pretend they never happened, a better approach is to learn from them.

Picture yourself in the midst of the hardest day in that season of your life. Now see the Lord standing right next to you, because He was.

Prayerfully reflect on the following questions: Are there unresolved feelings of guilt or resentment you haven't dealt with? Are there fears that linger as you enter those scenes in your mind? Do you see yourself acting against your conscience, doing what you wish you wouldn't? What is your biggest weaknesses in that moment? What causes you to reach for that extra pig-in-a-blanket? When are you most likely to shove cookie after cookie in your mouth, without even realizing what you're doing? Who is your companion in crime? Who elbows you and reassures with a wink that another bite won't hurt?

Close your eyes and go back to the scene. Picture yourself right there, in the midst of the hardest day in that season of your life. Now see the Lord standing right next to you, because He was. Whether we see and feel Him or not, God never leaves us. See yourself standing next to that buffet table or leaning over that toilet, and see the Good Shepherd right by your side.

What would He have said to you in that moment, if you had taken a moment to listen? What door of escape did He provide for you that you ignored? (Or maybe, in a moment of sheer obedience, you lunged for it and escaped temptation!)

As hard as it can be to go back to these moments, we learn so much from recognizing that God was right there with us. Often in Scripture, we see men and women of God affirm God's presence with them in the darkest seasons. David writes that the Lord is by him whether in the darkest valley (Psalm 23:4), in the quiet morning, or in the loneliest places of the world: "If I take the wings of the morning and dwell in the uttermost parts of the sea, even there your hand shall lead me, and your right hand shall hold me" (Psalm 139:9–10 ESV).

Rather than stuff down painful memories, we can recognize God's tender love and care for us even there, so that we can learn how to live victoriously moving forward.

Anticipate Future Struggles

With transitions you can anticipate, it helps to plan for changes before you're confronted with them. Review the chapters on spiritual disciplines and think of ways you can keep food in its proper place while finding joy and satisfaction in Jesus.

Spend some time with the Lord and prayerfully answer the following questions: What are the unique challenges you're going to face? How can you carve out time to spend with God so you're daily filled to overflowing with joy, peace, and hope? Which social engagements are most likely to present temptations to return to former food habits? Who's likely to encourage you to indulge in gluttonous behavior? How can you respond to that person in a gentle and firm way? Who can you ask to keep you accountable in your spiritually filling habits? Which magazines, websites, or outlets do you need to avoid so that you're getting healthy input in your life?

If you're planning a cross-country move, think about how you're going to handle meals during the transition. Plan a few healthy snacks when you can't find your pots and pans amid the labyrinth of half-packed boxes. Think about which kitchen staples you need on hand to start cooking healthy meals at your new place. Give yourself lots of grace during this high-stress transition, but also circle a date on the calendar when you'd like to have settled back into a new normal. Plan a check-in with the Lord at that point, and ask Him to show you any thought or eating patterns you've picked up that you need to surrender to Him.

Adapt to Your New Season

As humans, we're constantly changing, and so are our circumstances. As we evaluate our situation, it's important to stay flexible and adapt. What worked last year may not work this year. And that's okay, because life is a journey, and sometimes that takes twists and turns (as cheesy as that sounds). So in every season of life, we need to pray for victory, make a plan, be quick to obey, and reflect on our journey.

Pray for Victory

This step is so obvious it almost goes without saying, but for all that, we often forget to ask the Spirit of God to help us navigate these seasons that leave us feeling vulnerable. How often do we head into a party or gathering with trepidation, but don't ask the Lord to guide us? We just take a deep breath and hope for the best, and then later wonder what went wrong when we ate that fifth cookie.

We are told in Scripture to not lean on our own understanding or strength but rather to trust in the Lord with *all* our heart. What does this look like when it comes to the appetizer platters at a party? What kinds of things should we pray for in preparation for these seasons?

Self-control

As we've already seen, self-control is the fruit of the Spirit working in us. We need His help to rein in our cravings just as much as we need His help to quiet the incessant calorie counting and food comparison. Ask God to help you practice self-control as you walk into every situation.

Wisdom

So much of life is made up of little choices, and those have a way of snowballing into habits. Ask the Lord to give you wisdom to make the right choice every time, and trust that He will do so. As James reassures us, "If you need wisdom, ask our generous God, and he will give it to you. He will not rebuke you for asking. But when you ask him, be sure that your faith is in God alone. Do not waver, for a person with divided loyalty is as unsettled as a wave of the sea that is blown and tossed by the wind" (James 1:5–6 NLT). As you make a habit of asking for wisdom and help in the little decisions, you'll recognize

divine assistance in the littlest things. In that
moment, pause to thank Him for His help.
You'll be more likely to ask for help again if
you recognize that you received it when you
asked last time.

Godly entourage

If you've ever gone into a situation with the
best of intentions only to be pressured by
peers to indulge, you know the power of
persuasion. Scripture speaks to this as well,
and it's even in the context of food. Those
who don't have an eternal perspective in their
lives, who don't eat and drink for the glory of
God, are more likely to encourage you to eat
and drink whatever you want because "you
only live once." But that kind of "encouragement" will quickly dissolve your best resolutions (1 Corinthians 15:33). Instead, pray for
godly friends who will remind you of the
truths you've learned in your journey and
will lovingly keep you accountable every step
of the way. These are the friends who will
celebrate your victories with you and help lift
you when you stumble—just as you can lift
them and celebrate their victories with them.

Remember that you're not meant to fight this battle alone.
The Holy Spirit stands by, ready to help in our time of need.

Make a Plan

As you prayerfully consider the obstacles that you're likely to face in this season of your life, make a plan to overcome them. Be proactive about walking in obedience to the Lord instead of caving to temptation, by knowing how you're going to react when faced with a difficult situation. Some ideas are to write in your journal, review your food addiction Scripture memory cards, call a friend or trusted mentor, listen to worship music, write a letter to a persecuted brother or sister, clean out a closet and donate items to a relief organization, take a prayer walk around your neighborhood, read the Bible, read a devotional, drink a glass of water with lemon and reflect on John 7:37–39. And add your own ideas to this list!

Be Quick to Obey

A plan is useless without follow-through. But when followed closely, it can become the road map to navigating these seasons with their unique twists and turns.

The next time you're faced with a food temptation, implement the action step you committed to. As you partner with the Spirit of God to walk in obedience, you will notice gentle nudges in the right direction. *Be quick to obey.* Don't allow yourself to rationalize why you'll make an exception *just this time.* Allow the *The goal is progress, not perfection.* Spirit to lead you in obedience, and if that includes a deviation from the plan you settled on beforehand, you'll sense that in your spirit if you're in tune with Him.

Remember that the point here has never merely been shedding pounds. Our purpose is a deeper relationship with the Lord and these seemingly insignificant acts of obedience—stepping away from the table—enrich your relationship with God when they're done in partnership with Him. Keep your ear open to what the Lord has to say to you every step of the way, and be quick to obey.

Reflect on Your Journey

Have regular times of checking in with the Lord. Set aside a regular time each week when you can prayerfully reflect on the past days and evaluate whether or not your plan is working.

Celebrate victories when you were quick to obey the Spirit and experienced a breakthrough. Recognize these as victories and praise God for rescuing you. Have a dance party, like David (2 Samuel 6:14), and celebrate these steps of transformation because it means God is doing a new thing in your life. That's huge!

Think about the times you've broken your food boundaries in the past week. What doors had God opened to help you escape temptation that you ignored? Confess the times you failed to obey, and commit yourself to walk closely to God in similar situations. Ask for discernment as you reflect on "failures" to learn from them and obey in the future.

Worship God for His steadfast love and enduring character despite how often we fail. Rejoice in the salvation that is yours in Christ Jesus. Use every opportunity to draw closer to Him.

You've probably heard this before but the goal is progress, not perfection. Finding satisfaction in God is a journey that we continue to travel throughout our lives. New seasons in life don't have to trip us up or cause us to relapse into old habits or make new bad habits. Whether we're just now moving away to college or facing an empty nest or anything in between, each new season can mark the beginning of deeper transformation in our lives, as we discover new areas of our lives to bow before God and allow Him to mold us into the image of His Son.

As the story goes, I lost thirty pounds of that baby weight in the first month. (It sure does help that my baby weighed almost nine pounds. Goodness!) I'm writing this three months postpartum, and I'm not going to lie: I'm counting the days until I can fit into my pre-maternity clothes. But even though I'm tempted to adopt extreme diets to hurry this process along, I'm reminding myself that the point of this journey is not primarily to lose weight—it's to experience deeper heart transformation as I yield my life to Christ in this new season of my life.

And as I find joy in God during the midnight feedings and the afternoon cravings, He finds great delight in me—and in you too as you seek Him.

Digest the Truth

(for individual or group response)

1. What are some seasons of life you've already been through? What do you anticipate facing in the near future?

2. Look again at the section Evaluate Your Current Situation on pages 223–25. Are there things in your daily life you have not been aware of before that could trip you up?

3. How might your known triggers affect how you deal with a change in life, big or small? Be as specific as you can.

4. What steps can you take to remain healthy during major changes in life?

Bonus Online Content

Download the worksheet "Journaling Questions to Jump-Start Change" at http://www.thefull.life/jumpstart-change.

Afterword

Standing at the kitchen sink recently, I scrubbed pots while sharing with a friend my yearlong journey that God had taken me on. I told her the highlights and the low points, and she listened with rapt attention.

When I finished, she asked, "But would you say you've overcome food addiction completely?"

I sat back on my heels, elbow deep in soapsuds and pondered the question.

I am in a different place today than I was two years ago, but I still have a long way to go. And even having written down the lessons I've learned along the way, I'm still finding that I need to go back and relearn them. Paul speaks to this issue when he encourages believers, "If you think you are standing firm, be careful that you don't fall!" (1 Corinthians 10:12). There is great wisdom in acknowledging our vulnerability to the things that have caused us to stumble in the past, but we do not have to live in fear of being controlled by those things.

Jesus has set me free from food fixation, and He continues to free me every day. As you've journeyed with me through this book, I hope you can say the same. He breaks the chains that bind us, takes away the shame that cripples us, and frees us to live in freedom. He calls us to find comfort and satisfaction in Him alone, and He fills us to the measure with all the fullness of God. He looks to us and whispers, "You are Mine, and I would fill you to overflowing with riches you cannot even fathom, if you'd let Me, from this day on into eternity." So we choose daily whether to respond to His call or slink back to the empty promises of food idols. And when we say yes to God, He gives us more than we could have asked for or imagined.

This walk on earth becomes the training grounds for an eternity spent glorifying God and enjoying Him forever. And one day we will see Him face to face, unhindered by our sinful nature, free to worship in our newly-resurrected bodies. We will join the millions of believers who have overcome sin and death by the blood of the Lamb and the word of their testimony, singing together with the angels,

> Worthy is the Lamb, who was slain,
> to receive power and wealth and wisdom and strength
> and honor and glory and praise! . . .
> To him who sits on the throne and to the Lamb
> be praise and honor and glory and power,
> for ever and ever! (Revelation 5:12–13)

Until then, we have the privilege of inviting more and more people to taste and see that the Lord is good, to give up the empty food trappings that don't satisfy and find fullness in Jesus. And if that's you at the end of this book, then, what are you waiting for? Come on!

The Spirit and the bride say, "Come!" And let the one who hears say, "Come!" Let the one who is thirsty come; and let the one who wishes take the free gift of the water of life. (Revelation 22:17)

Bonus Online Content

Watch Asheritah share encouragement to keep living The Full Life as well as what you can do now that you've finished this book at http://www.thefull.life/afterword.

Bonus Section

The Food-Fixation Assessment

Twenty Verses to Overcome Food Fixation

A Pastor's Comment

The Food-Fixation Assessment

Whether our weakness is skinny lattes, French fries, or Oreos, many of us feel consumed with thoughts and longings for food. But how do we know when this preoccupation has become a *food fixation?* Choose the scenario below that best represents you then use the ten statements to assess yourself.

Scenario #1:

After a hard day, do you reward yourself with food? If yes, take the comfort food fixation assessment below. Read the following statements and honestly rate how well they describe you, with 1 being "never," and 5 being "constantly."

_____ 1. I tell myself, "I'll start my diet tomorrow."

_____ 2. I go to bed regretting what I ate that day.

_____ 3. I feel guilty when I indulge in a dessert.

_____ 4. I try to give up certain unhealthy foods but feel like I can't live without them.

_____ 5. I feel hopeless about my relationship with food.

_____ 6. I keep eating certain foods even though I'm no longer hungry.

_____ 7. I eat what I crave regardless of whether it's good for me or not.

_____ 8. I'm more likely to eat to escape my feelings than pray about them.

_____9. I feel trapped in a cycle of dieting and overeating.

_____10. How closely I follow my eating plan affects whether I feel good or bad about myself.

Scenario #2:

When eating outside your home, do you find it hard not to think and talk about what's in your food? If yes, take the healthy food fixation assessment below. Read the following statements and honestly rate how well they describe you, with 1 being "never," and 5 being "constantly."

_____1. When I get together with friends, we talk about the latest diets or food trends.

_____2. Friends have told me that I take my healthy eating plan too seriously.

_____3. I can't travel without bringing along my own healthy food.

_____4. I think less of people who don't value healthy eating as much as I do.

_____5. I talk to my friends more about food than I do about Jesus.

_____6. I worry that if I don't eat the right way, I'm going to suffer from serious diseases.

_____7. I tell my friends how important it is to eat the right way—whether they want to hear it or not.

_____8. How closely I follow my eating plan affects whether I feel good or bad about myself.

_____9. I feel guilty when I indulge in a dessert.

_____10. I'm more likely to look up healthy recipes and posts on Pinterest than I am to look up Scripture.

Now determine your total score by adding all of your ratings together.

Scores of 10–19:

Food is no big deal to you. To you, food is simply fuel for your body, and you don't spend too much time worrying about it. If someone offers you a treat, you can take a bite or two and walk away without a second thought. You try to eat healthy but don't stress too much about controlling every bite you eat. You may have a hard time understanding why other people struggle with their food choices. While you may not have a food fixation, chances are you know someone who does.

Scores of 20–34:

Food can sometimes dominate your thoughts, but you also have times when food fades into the background and you discover the beauty of life without food struggles. You find that certain situations trigger an obsession with food and you're not always sure how to handle those situations to minimize their impact on your thought life. While food fixation may not be your biggest worry right now, learning God's perspective on food will help you break the power of food in your life and set you free to taste and see that God is better even than chocolate cake.

Scores of 35–50:

You have a love-hate relationship with food, and dislike the fact that your food choices control you. You often feel that your life revolves around your food choices, consuming energy that should be going to your spiritual life, work, and family. You've tried countless plans to break free from your bondage to food, but you still feel enslaved and hopeless. This book will help you engage the spiritual battle that's affecting not only your waistline but also your lifeline to God, helping you experience deeper intimacy with God, gain a renewed sense of purpose, and enjoy good food.

Twenty Verses to
Overcome Food Fixation

So whether you eat or drink or whatever you do, do it all for
the glory of God. —1 Corinthians 10:31

Unless the Lord builds the house, the builders labor in vain.
. . . In vain you rise early and stay up late, toiling for food to
eat—for he grants sleep to those he loves. —Psalm 127:1–2

You have made your way around this hill country long
enough; now turn north. —Deuteronomy 2:3

We demolish arguments and every pretension that sets itself
up against the knowledge of God, and we take captive every
thought to make it obedient to Christ. —2 Corinthians 10:5

But he said to me, "My grace is sufficient for you, for my power
is made perfect in weakness." Therefore I will boast all the
more gladly about my weaknesses, so that Christ's power may
rest on me. . . . For when I am weak, then I am strong.
—2 Corinthians 12:9–10

Blessed are those whose strength is in you. . . . They go from
strength to strength, till each appears before God in Zion.
—Psalm 84:5,7

He has delivered us from the domain of darkness and transferred us to the kingdom of his beloved Son, in whom we have
redemption, the forgiveness of sins. —Colossians 1:13–14 ESV

Do you not know that your bodies are temples of the Holy Spirit, who is in you, whom you have received from God? You are not your own. —1 Corinthians 6:19

Therefore put on the full armor of God. . . . Stand firm then, with the belt of truth . . . the breastplate of righteousness . . . the gospel of peace . . . the shield of faith . . . the helmet of salvation and the sword of the Spirit, which is the word of God. And pray in the Spirit on all occasions with all kinds of prayers and requests. —Ephesians 6:13–18

"I have the right to do anything" . . .—but not everything is beneficial.
"I have the right to do anything"—but I will not be mastered by anything. —1 Corinthians 6:12

The heart is deceitful above all things and beyond cure. Who can understand it? "I the Lord search the heart and examine the mind, to reward each person according to their conduct, according to what their deeds deserve." —Jeremiah 17:9–10

You prepare a table before me in the presence of my enemies. You anoint my head with oil; my cup overflows. —Psalm 23:5

No temptation has overtaken you except what is common to mankind. And God is faithful; he will not let you be tempted beyond what you can bear. But when you are tempted, he will also provide a way out so that you can endure it.
—1 Corinthians 10:13–14

So if the Son sets you free, you will be free indeed. —John 8:36

Those who feel free to eat anything must not look down on those who don't. And those who don't eat certain foods must not condemn those who do, for God has accepted them. —Romans 14:3–5 NLT

See, I have placed before you an open door that no one can shut. —Revelation 3:8

Then he said to them all: "Whoever wants to be my disciple must deny themselves and take up their cross daily and follow me." —Luke 9:23

Then Jesus declared, "I am the bread of life. Whoever comes to me will never go hungry, and whoever believes in me will never be thirsty." —John 6:35

Just as you used to offer yourselves as slaves to impurity and to ever-increasing wickedness, so now offer yourselves as slaves to righteousness leading to holiness. —Romans 6:19

The thief comes only to steal and kill and destroy; I have come that they may have life, and have it to the full. —John 10:10

A Pastor's Comment

I asked my pastor the following question: "Do our food struggles influence our witness to the onlooking unbelieving world? If so, in what way, and how can we better testify to the satisfaction found in Jesus?"

Here is his response:

I believe that food fixation, gluttony, and obesity are all distinct issues of the soul, sometimes deeply interrelated but not necessarily so. But the question of how these influence our witness to the world raises the issues of personal responsibility as well as pastoral leadership.

I think this issue of obesity in the church is becoming increasingly important to the testimony of Christ entrusted to the church in our twenty-first century Western culture. Our culture insists that an individual has ultimate authority over his or her body. The crux of most of our hot-button social issues are founded on the premise "My body is mine to command; it is my right to do so; it is my choice to make; it is my preference to dictate." That is the foundation of the debate over abortion, sexual activity before marriage, homosexuality, sexual identity, euthanasia . . . and the list goes on!

As long as I don't hurt another (so the argument goes), what right does God have to tell me what I should or should not do with my body? And we who are believers in the God who made our bodies respond in humility, "He has every right." Yet we have a tendency to exclude the issue of how our sinful use of food impacts our bodies. And we have the tendency to ignore gluttony and the potential obesity that results as being irrelevant (intentionally or not). To be sure, those who hear us talk about God's rights in all the other body-behavior categories notice the inconsistency (or hypocrisy) and are quick to point it out. For all practical purposes, we may well be reinforcing the ever-increasing premise of "my body, my right, my preference," and undermining the message we are trying to proclaim.

Therefore, this issue of obesity in the church (which is very real) does have a direct impact on how we testify to God's command on our lives, our call to disciple others in Christ, and our call to others who need to know the Creator God who has the right to tell us how we handle our bodies. After all, Paul invites us several times in various ways to follow his example (see 1 Corinthians 4:16, 11:1; Philippians 3:17, 4:19; 1 Thessalonians 1:6; 2 Thessalonians 3:9). It is at the heart of the meaning of discipleship, and those who would lead must see this issue with ever-increasing awareness in our culture, inside and outside the church.

And as with all the other issues with which the church struggles, we should speak with love, and speak with grace, and speak with clarity as we lead by example with God's mercy in our own lives.

MIKE CASTELLI
Lead Pastor
The Chapel in Green

Notes

Chapter 1: Know That Calories Aren't the Enemy

1. Elyse Fitzpatrick, *Love to Eat, Hate to Eat: Breaking the Bondage of Destructive Eating Habits* (Eugene, OR: Harvest House, 1999), 17.

2. Herbert Lockyer, "Glutton," *Nelson's Illustrated Bible Dictionary* (Nashville: Thomas Nelson, 1986), 448.

3. Fitzpatrick, *Love to Eat, Hate to Eat,* 101.

4. Leslie Ludy, *The Set-Apart Woman: God's Invitation to Sacred Living* (Colorado Springs: NavPress, 2015), 142–43.

5. Annie Downs, *Looking for Lovely: Collecting the Moments That Matter* (Nashville: B&H Publishing Group, 2016), 37.

6. C. L. Ogden, M. D. Carroll, H. G. Lawman, C. D. Fryar, D. Kruszon-Moran, B. K. Kit, and K. M. Flegal. (2016). "Trends in obesity prevalence among children and adolescents in the United States, 1988–1994 through 2013–2014." *JAMA*, 315(21), 2292–99, http://frac.org/initiatives/hunger-and-obesity/obesity-in-the-us/.

7. Amanda L. Chan, "Prescription Drugs: 7 Out of 10 Americans Take At Least One, Study Finds." *The Huffington Post.* TheHuffingtonPost.com. http://www.huffingtonpost.com/2013/06/19/prescription-drugs-prevalence-americans_n_3466801.html.

8. Beth Moore, *Praying God's Word: Breaking Free from Spiritual Strongholds* (Nashville: B&H, 2000), 3.

9. Jennie Allen, "Disciple a Generation" (speech at IF: Gathering Local Leaders Conference), accessed on Right Now Media.

Chapter 2: Dress for Success

1. Neal D. Barnard and Joanne Stepaniak, *Breaking the Food Seduction: The Hidden Reasons Behind Food Cravings—and 7 Steps to End Them Naturally* (New York: St. Martin's Press, 2003), 9.

2. Anne Katherine, *Anatomy of a Food Addiction: The Brain Chemistry of Overeating* (Carlsbad, CA: Gurze Books, 1996), 26.

3. Kathleen DesMaisons, *The Sugar Addict's Total Recovery Program* (New York: Ballantine Pub Group, 2000), 151.

4. Lysa TerKeurst, *Made to Crave: Satisfying Your Deepest Desire with God, Not Food* (Grand Rapids: Zondervan, 2010), 19.

5. Kenneth L. Barker and Donald W. Burdick, "Study Note on Isaiah 11:5" in *Zondervan NIV Study Bible* (Grand Rapids: Zondervan, 2002).

Chapter 3: Choose Truth Over Lies

1. Brian Wansink, *Mindless Eating: Why We Eat More Than We Think* (New York: Bantam Books, 2006), 72.

Chapter 4: Stir Up a Holy Hunger

1. Elyse Fitzpatrick, *Love to Eat, Hate to Eat* (Eugene, OR: Harvest House, 1999), 77.

2. Ibid., 74.

3. Beth Moore, *Praying God's Word: Breaking Free from Spiritual Strongholds* (Nashville: B&H, 2000), 6.

4. Amy Carmichael, "Crooked Patterns," *God's Missionary* (Fort Washington: Christian Literature Crusade, 1997), 15.

5. John Piper, *A Hunger for God: Desiring God through Fasting and Prayer* (Wheaton: Crossway Books, 1997), 23.

6. Thomas Watson, *The Beatitudes: An Exposition of Matthew 5:1–12,* as quoted in Leslie Ludy, *The Set-Apart Woman* (Colorado Springs: NavPress, 2015), 109.

7. For more of Monica's story, go to www.monicaswanson.com.

Chapter 5: Experience the Power of Fasting

1. Richard Foster, *Celebration of Discipline* (San Francisco: Harper & Row, 1988), 48–52.

2. Don Whitney, *Spiritual Disciplines for the Christian Life* (Colorado Springs: NavPress, 2014), 200–214. According to Whitney, all the following are appropriate reasons to fast:

To strengthen prayer (Ezra 8:23; Joel 2:13; Acts 13:3)

To seek God's guidance (Judges 20:16; Acts 14:23)

To express grief (1 Samuel 31:13; 2 Samuel 1:11–12)

To seek deliverance or protection (2 Chronicles 20:3–4; Ezra 8:21–23)

To express repentance and return to God (1 Samuel 7:6; Jonah 3:5–8)

To humble oneself before God (1 Kings 21:27–29; Psalm 35:13)

To express concern for the work of God (Nehemiah 1:3–4; Daniel 9:3)

To minister to the needs of others (Isaiah 58:3–7)

To overcome temptation and dedicate yourself to God (Matthew 4:1–11)

To express love and worship to God (Luke 2:37)

3. John Piper, *A Hunger for God* (Wheaton, IL: Crossway, 2013), 24.

4. Quoted by Joni Eareckson Tada, "When Jesus Is All You Have," Joni and Friends, July 28, 2006, http://www.joniandfriends.org/radio/5-minute/when-jesus-all-you-have/.

5. David Mathis, "Fasting for Beginners," Desiring God, August 26, 2015, http://www.desiringgod.org/articles/fasting-for-beginners.

Chapter 6: Feast on God's Word

1. Jim Cymbala, "Driven to Kindness," The Brooklyn Tabernacle Blogs (blog), November 21, 2015, http://blog.brooklyntabernacle.org/jim_cymbala/2015/11/21/driven-to-kindness-part-4/.

2. Jen Wilkin, *Women of the Word: How to Study the Bible with Both Our Hearts and Our Minds* (Wheaton, IL: Crossway, 2014), 33.

3. Leland Wang, "No Bible, No Breakfast," Joyful Heart Renewal Ministries, http://www.joyfulheart.com/maturity/no-bible-no-breakfast.htm.

4. For a fuller explanation of the FEAST method, visit http://www.onethingalone.com/feast.

5. An excellent resource is *His Word in My Heart: Memorizing Scripture for a Closer Walk with God* by Janet Pope (Chicago: Moody, 2013).

6. D. L. Moody, *Notes from My Bible and Thoughts from My Library* (Grand Rapids: Baker, 1979), 110.

Chapter 7: Discover Your Triggers

1. Susan McQuillan, "Food Triggers" in *Breaking the Bonds of Food Addiction* (New York: Alpha, 2004), Kindle edition.

2. Barb Raveling, *I Deserve a Donut (And Other Lies That Make You Eat)* (Truthway Press, 2013), Kindle edition.

3. Bill Hull, quoted in Elizabeth George, *Life Management for Busy Women* (Eugene, OR: Harvest House, 2002), 88.

4. Linda Dillow, *Satisfy My Thirsty Soul: For I Am Desperate for Your Presence* (Colorado Springs: NavPress, 2007), 19.

Chapter 8: Celebrate the Gift of Food

1. *The Shorter Catechism* as quoted in G. I. Williamson, *The Shorter Catechism* (Nutley, NJ: Presbyterian and Reformed Pub. Co, 1970), 1.

2. Charles John Ellicott, "1 Timothy 4:5," in *The Pastoral Epistles of St.*

Paul (London: Cassell, 1870), BibleHub.com/commentaries/ellicott/1_timothy/4.htm.

3. Robert Jamieson, A. R. Fausset, and David Brown, "1 Timothy 4:5," in *A Commentary Critical, Practical and Explanatory, on the Old and New Testaments* (New York: F.H. Revell), http://biblehub.com/commentaries/jfb/1_timothy/4.htm.

4. Lysa TerKeurst, *Made to Crave: Satisfying Your Deepest Desire with God, Not Food* (Grand Rapids: Zondervan, 2010), 19.

5. Elyse Fitzpatrick, *Love to Eat, Hate to Eat* (Eugene, OR: Harvest House, 1999), 111.

6. "NIH Study Sheds Light on How to Reset the Addicted Brain," National Institutes of Health, April 3, 2013, https://www.nih.gov/newsevents/news-releases/nih-study-sheds-light-how-reset-addicted-brain.

Chapter 9: Run to Win

1. Beth Moore, *Praying God's Word: Breaking Free from Spiritual Strongholds* (Nashville: B&H, 2009), 128.

2. If you're not sure if you have a personal relationship with Jesus, He wants you to have assurance of your salvation. Learn how you can be forgiven of your sins and live with Him forever at www.onethingalone.com/salvation.

3. In the Old Testament book of Leviticus, Israel's priests were instructed to offer animals as sacrifices to atone for the people's sins. God required that these sacrificial animals be without any blemish, and there were strict regulations regarding these sacrifices. These sin offerings pointed the people to the ultimate sacrifice: Jesus Christ, the spotless Lamb of God, who took our sins upon Himself and secured for us God's forgiveness and eternal salvation.

4. Christine Caine, *Unashamed: Drop the Baggage, Pick up Your Freedom, Fulfill Your Destiny* (Grand Rapids: Zondervan, 2016), Kindle edition.

5. Elizabeth Esther, *Spiritual Sobriety: Stumbling Back to Faith When Good Religion Goes Bad* (New York: Convergent Books, 2016), 162–63.

Chapter 10. Embrace the Grace of Community

1. A 2011 Northwestern University study tracking 2,433 men and women for eighteen years found that young adults who attend church or a bible study once a week are 50 percent more likely to be obese. See Maria Paul, "Religious Young Adults Become Obese by Middle Age," Northwestern University, March 23, 2011, http://www.northwestern.edu/newscenter/stories/2011/03/religious-young-adults-obese.html.

See also Eryn Sun, "Firm Faith, Fat Body?" Christian Post, March 24, 2011, http://www.christianpost.com/news/firm-faith-fat-body-study-finds-high-rate-of-obesity-among-religious-49568/#Zo7zlJFhsEbB-PscP.99 and Scott Stoll, "Fat in Church," Fox News, January 04, 2013, http://www.foxnews.com/opinion/2012/06/03/obesity-epidemic-in-america-churches.html. nydailynews.com/life-style/health/one-third-clergy-members-obese-study-article-1.2075168.

2. http://biblehub.com/greek/810.htm.

3. Data from The World Bank, accessed June 25, 2016, http://data.worldbank.org/indicator/SP.POP.TOTL

4. Frank Newport, "In U.S., Four in 10 Report Attending Church in Last Week," Gallup, December 24, 2013, http://www.gallup.com/poll/166613/four-report-attending-church-last-week.aspx.

5. Bureau of Labor Statistics, "Consumer Expenditures 2014," September 3, 2015, http://www.bls.gov/news.release/pdf/cesan.pdf.

6. "Become a Full Life Monthly Partner," LeSEA Global Feed the Hungry, https://feedthehungry.org/our-impact/full-life-monthly-partners/.

7. David Fisher, interview by author, June 1, 2016.

8. "Pastor Sees Healthy Lifestyle as Act of Worship," Baptist Standard, March 17, 2011, https://www.baptiststandard.com/news/texas/12319-pastor-sees-healthy-lifestyle-as-act-of-worship.

Chapter 11: Serve with Food

1. "Koinonia," Bible Study Tools, http://www.biblestudytools.com/lexicons/greek/nas/koinonia.html.

2. Shauna Niequist, Bread and Wine: A Love Letter to Live around the Table with Recipes (Grand Rapids: Zondervan, 2013), 114.

3. The bestselling The 5 Love Languages: The Secret to Love That Lasts by Gary Chapman is an amazing and practical book explaining how we each have different ways of giving and receiving love. The five love languages are words of affirmation, gifts, quality time, acts of service, physical touch. www.5lovelanguages.com.

Chapter 12: Navigate Seasons of Change

1. These questions were inspired by Barb Raveling's excellent book I Deserve a Donut.

Acknowledgments

Lord, thank You for stirring in me a hunger for You. You put this message in my heart, gave strength to my weary mama limbs to write, and opened doors for me to walk through. This is all from You and through You and for You. Nothing is sweeter than You.

Iubitul meu Flaviu, thank you for speaking words of life over me in the darkest nights and for creating room for me to create. It's always better when we're together. And to Carissa and Amelia, thank you for all the giggles and snuggles after a long day of work. May you grow to discover your deepest joy and satisfaction in the Jesus your mama and *tata* love so dearly. To my in-laws, thank you for tenderly caring for our precious girls while I wrote this book.

Mom, you called out the talent you saw in me from a young age before anyone else did. And Dad, you cultivated in me a love for words. Thank you both for raising me in fear and love of God, and also passing on your love for good food. So many fun memories around both campfires and linen-covered tables!

Tawny, thank you for guiding me through the unknowns of the publishing world and always taking time. Always. You're the best agent a writer could hope for. Ingrid, thank you for listening to my heart and taking a chance on this young writer. You caught my vision and championed this message until it reached the world. Pam, you took a disjointed and wordy manuscript and edited it into a beautiful book. Thank you. And to Ashley, Randall, Connor, Eric, and the rest of the Moody team—you guys rock. Seriously, I'm beyond thrilled to launch this book with you all.

To Ana, Laura, Jennifer, Sara, Katie, Joanna, Jenn, Monica, and Pastor Dave, thank you for trusting me with your stories. You brought a richness and dimension to this narrative that shows *anyone* can have as much of Jesus as they want, and I can't help but think that our stories mingle together into a pleasing aroma to Him.

To Wendy, Kate, Amy, Katie, Brittany, Kelly, and so many other writer friends, thank you for traveling this road with me. Truly, there is no room for competition when we link arms to move God's kingdom forward. What a precious gift your friendship is to me!

To Carmen, Sara, and my dear prayer warriors, thank you from the bottom of my heart for your prayer covering. How many times did I send out an SOS and you all came rushing in to ask for God to move mightily? And move mightily He did. Thank you, dear sisters for praying this book into being and holding up my arms when they were weak. And Pastor Mike, thank you for your expert critique; this book is so much better thanks to your gentle shepherding.

To my Green Chapel family, thank you for letting me do life alongside you. Thank you for serving our family in a million little ways, and thank you for allowing us to serve you as well. A writer is only as good as the community surrounding her, pouring into her, and reminding her that she is a human being before doing anything else. You are my people.

To my One Thing Alone readers, thank you for your encouragement and feedback. Your emails and messages saying

"Me too!" were the impetus to push forward through stretches of unproductive days to bring forth this message.

And to you, gentle reader, thank you for trusting me to walk alongside you in this journey toward the full life in Jesus. We're in this together, you and I, and we keep pressing onward as we run this race to the finish. I'd love to hear how God is working in your life and pray for you as you journey forward. Feel free to email me at asheritah@onethingalone.com.